The Book Collecting Practices of Black Magazine Editors

by Thomas Weissinger

Litwin Books
Sacramento, CA

Copyright 2014 Thomas Weissinger

Published in 2014 by Litwin Books

Litwin Books
PO Box 188784
Sacramento, CA 95818

http://litwinbooks.com/

This book is printed on acid-free, sustainably-sourced paper.

Library of Congress Cataloging-in-Publication Data

Weissinger, Thomas.
 The book collecting practices of Black magazine editors / Thomas Weissinger.
   pages cm
 Summary: "Focuses on the collecting habits and personal libraries of the editors three Black magazines: Ben Burns, Era Bell Thompson, and Tom Dent"-- Provided by publisher.
 Includes bibliographical references and index.
 ISBN 978-1-936117-63-5 (acid-free paper)
  1. African American book collectors--Biography. 2. Periodical editors--United States--Biography. 3. Burns, Ben--Library. 4. Thompson, Era Bell--Library. 5. Dent, Thomas C.--Library. 6. Private libraries--United States. 7. African American academic libraries. 8. Libraries--Special collections--African Americans. 9. African Americans--Bibliography--Methodology. 10. African American periodicals--History--20th century. I. Title.
 Z989.A1W45 2014
 027'.108996073--dc23
            2014002547

Table of Contents

1   Introduction

5   **Chapter 1**
        Personal Libraries: From Comprehensive
        to Working Libraries

15   **Chapter 2**
        Stances on Race Equality

27   **Chapter 3**
        Experiences in Book Collecting: A Bibliographic Essay

55   **Chapter 4**
        Text Network Analysis

Introduction

The personal libraries of influential black bibliophiles often became the foundations of African American rare book and special collections libraries. In the words of Jesse Carney Smith, Fisk University Librarian and authority on black bibliography, "black collections in libraries ... have felt the influence of persons such as Arthur A. Schomburg, Carl Van Vechten, Langston Hughes, and Arthur Spingarn, either through materials which they presented to these libraries to enrich their collection or through the purchase of collections which they assembled. Such persons have therefore had a marked effect on the development of notable collections of black literature." Their personal libraries have been pivotal to establishing major collections at Howard University, the New York Public Library, the Library of Congress, the Atlanta University Center, and Fisk University, and others, to name a few. Although primarily about African American life and culture, the personal libraries of black bibliophiles also included books about other parts of the African diaspora.[1]

Authorities such as Jessie Carney Smith also believe more studies about the development of special black collections are necessary. She writes that:

> The historical development of special black collections that have been assembled and subsequently housed in American libraries would make interesting study. Doubtless, the patterns of their development would vary, yet one common element in their background would be the sheer love of books, manuscripts, or archives that someone possessed. ...This someone—this great collector—could have been Arthur Spingarn, Arthur Schomburg, W. E. B. Du Bois, Charles F. Heartman, Clarence Holte,

or Charles Blockson. Or, the collector could have been one whose name is little known, but who helped to preserve important an currently popular local history collections.²

Randall K. Burkett, Curator of African American Collections at Emory University, agrees with Smith, but takes the idea of researching the development of special black collections a step further, to researching the window they provide into the mind of the person who assembled them." Regarding the importance of research, Burkett writes:

> personal libraries of great intellectuals such as Carter Godwin Woodson, need to be preserved in their entirety. They are important, of course, for the rare books they contain. But they are equally important for the window they provide into the world of ideas, and into the mind of the person who assembled them... The library in its entirety suggests the intellectual universe from which an individual could draw in doing his or her own work."³

The shift from preserving important black personal libraries to reflecting on the use which their collectors made of them is an epiphany of sorts. It is a striking turn of thought regarding how black personal libraries are considered. This is certainly an under-studied aspect of black bibliography, one which the present work aims to address.

Two recent works, one an unpublished manuscript by Abdul Alkalimat, the other a co-authored article by Abdul Alkalimat and Ron Daniels, also show signs of a shift in thinking about black personal libraries. The two authors also are interested in the fact that such collections reflect the mindsets of individuals, but are on a somewhat different track. They are chiefly concerned about whose mindsets are reflected and whether there are safeguards against racist books in large digital collections. Alkalimat and Daniels have an interest in digitizing books from black special collections in order to accurately reflect black culture and counter racism. Their thoughts are discussed further in next chapter.⁴

The present study focuses on three black magazine editors. Ben Burns and Era Bell Thompson were editors of the *Negro Digest*, *Ebony*, and *Jet* magazines. Tom Dent edited *Umbra* and *Nkombo*, two important black literary magazines. As influential editors of the black press, these individuals disseminated information about black culture and social affairs on a national level. For instance, during the World War II the *Negro Digest* sold more than 150,000 issues a month, enabling the Johnson Publishing Company to move into expanded and improved facilities. Between 1949 and 1951 the *Negro Digest* sold as many as 100,000 issues each year. Comparing paid circulation figures for the first half of each year, *Ebony's* circulation increased from 324,930 in 1948 to 492,544 in 1954. In the early 1950s *Jet* exceeded the circulation of all other African American weeklies, selling 300,000 issues a week.[5] Circulation numbers for *Umbra* and *Nkombo* magazines are not available, but there is evidence that these were two of the most important literary magazines of the Black Arts Movement.[6]

This study will be of interest to librarians, library educators, bibliophiles, historians, laypersons, and students of American culture. Building upon prior research in black bibliography, the study examines the reasons why certain black press editors sought to assemble personal libraries of their own. It considers the effect of racial ideology on their collection building activities. The study takes a look at how the collections of the three bibliophiles are configured and what makes them useful. A mixed-methods approach is used for data analysis. Historical analysis based on primary and secondary sources is used to discern the racial ideologies and personal experiences of the book collectors. Text network analysis is used to analyze the structure and configuration of their personal libraries. Uncovered are the relations between important subjects and various forms and genre styles. These are prescriptive in nature and offer practical guidance in terms of how to build functional African American personal libraries.

Notes

1. Smith, Jessie Carney. *Black Academic Libraries and Research Collections: An Historical Survey.* Westport, CT: Greenwood Press, 1977, p.166.

2. Smith, Jessie Carney. "An Overview, including the Special Collections at Fisk University." In Sinnette, Elinor Des Verney, W. Paul Coates and Thomas C. Battle, eds. *Black Bibliophiles and Collectors.* Washington DC: Howard University Press, 1990, p. 60.

3. Ibid., p. 157; and Burkett, Randall K., Pellom McDaniels, and Tiffany Gleason. *The Mind of Carter G. Woodson as Reflected in the Books He Owned, Read, & Published: A Catalog of the Library of Carter G. Woodson and the Association for the Study of African American Life and History.* Atlanta, GA: Emory University, 2006), p. 8.

4. Alkalimat, Abdul. "African American Bibliography: The social construction of a literature of record," November, 2012, unpublished manuscript, p. 17; and Alkalimat, Abdul and Ronald Bailey. "From Black to eBlack: The Digital Transformation of Black Studies Pedagogy." *Fire!!!: The Multimedia Journal of Black Studies*, vol. 1, no. 1.

5. For *Negro Digest* subscription numbers see Burns, Ben. *Nitty Gritty: A White Editor in Black Journalism.* Jackson, MS: University Press of Mississippi, 1996, p. 39; and *N. W. Ayer & Son's Directory: Newspapers and Periodicals* (Philadelphia: N. W. Ayer & Sons) annuals for 1949, 1950 and 1951, pages 1269, 1325 and 1327, respectively. For *Ebony* subscription numbers see the annuals for 1948, 1949, 1950, 1951, 1952, 1953 and 1954, pages 1258, 1269, 1325, 1327, 1333, 1338 and 1345, respectively. For *Jet* numbers see Burns, Ben. *Nitty Gritty*, p. 167.

6. Thomas, Lorenzo. "The Need to Speak: Tom Dent and the Shaping of a Black Aesthetic." *African American Review* 40.2 (2006): 327; Ibid., p. 330.; and Thomas, Lorenzo. Southern Black Aesthetics: the Case of Nkombo Magazine." *Mississippi Quarterly* 44 (Spring 1991): 143-150.

CHAPTER ONE

Personal Libraries: From Comprehensive to Working Libraries

The discussion about black heritage personal libraries often turns around the accomplishments of notable black bibliophiles, many of whom were mentioned in preceding paragraphs. The bibliophiles are revered for having discovered, unearthed, or preserved heretofore inaccessible truths about black heritage. They are revered for their scholarship and perseverance. One of Arthur Schomburg's biographers reasons that the early black bibliophiles were diligent because the societies in which they lived were skeptical about the intellectual ability of black people. The collectors, therefore, regarded their bibliophilia as a mission and commitment to disproving the skeptics. The personal libraries built by such bibliophiles filled a void at a time when scholarship by and about African Americans was inaccessible or overlooked.[1]

Illustrative of the respect bestowed on black bibliophiles is Hanes Walton, Jr.'s "To Clarence Holte: The Black Bibliophile Par Excellence." This is an acknowledgement prefacing Walton's book *Black Republicans: The Politics of the Black and Tans* (1975), which is about Reconstruction era politics in the South. Clarence Holte was a black advertising director, publisher, and esteemed book collector with one of the largest private collections of books on black history and culture. Some of Walton's tribute reads as follows:

> The word bibliophile means "one who loves books, especially for their binding and style." Mr. Holte is a bibliophile, but not in that sense. He is a seeker of the truth, a searcher in the Darkness for Light, and a groper in the backways, the byways and lowways for the Black Past. … a layman, like yourself—a man who earns his way outside of academia—contributes to

the growing intellectual wisdom, that Blacks are not without a past worth speaking of before the coming of the white man. … Alone, and without the comfort of cloistered academia, you have searched and found the truth, not its bindings or style. And the Clarence L. Holte Collection, like the Black Past, is second to none. …So, Clarence L. Holte, I salute you and place you with Woodson, Dubois, and Hansberry. In a way your commitment and insights are much greater than theirs—for they were partly motivated by their academic backgrounds—you rose from the masses, the "Soul" of Black people.[2]

Types of Black Bibliophile

There are many kinds of personal library and specificity is needed when bandying the phrase around. Personal libraries range from the general home library of miscellaneous titles, collections arranged around certain themes, and rare book collections. The general home library can be both aesthetically pleasing and/or a source of enlightenment. Aesthetically, such libraries certify a degree of accomplishment and literary refinement. As one writer puts it, "Why not put your most handsome sets and newest books where everyone will see them? After all books are beautiful furniture." In this same vein, "a choice collection of books can make an impression on those having an opportunity to peruse it."

In academia the value of personal working libraries is often associated with their usefulness to faculty research. The convenience of having source material nearby is important in the day-to-day work of researchers. Researchers buy books that they believe will be frequently used and if they are affordable.[3]

In a short article entitled "Professional and Amateur Collectors Indulge a Passion for Black History and Culture" (*Black Book Review*, February 28, 1996), Angela Ards lays out a schema describing the many kinds of book collector commonly known as "black bibliophiles." Four models of black bibliophile are identified, each with a different purpose for building personal libraries about African Americans. The purposes are collecting for posterity and legacy, collecting for knowledge, collecting for empowerment, and collecting for joy. Arthur Schomburg and Charles

Blockson are said to typify the first model.

Arthur Schomburg, the most well-known of the black bibliophiles, had amassed between 5,000 to 6,000 volumes when he sold his collection to the Carnegie Foundation in 1926. Among the rare material included in the collection are first editions of works by Phillis Wheatley and William Wells Brown, William Banneker's Almanac, and abolitionist sermons written by former slaves. Absorbe into the Schomburg personal library were books which formerly belonged to the Negro Society for Historical Research, an association founded by himself and newspaper columnist/editor John Edward Bruce. Also John Edward Bruce's collection was incorporated into Schomburg's as a donation by his widow when Bruce died in 1924. After its purchase by the Carnegie Foundation for $10,000, Schomburg's collection became the backbone for the Division of Negro History, Literature and Prints of the 135th Street Branch of the New York Public Library.[4]

Charles L. Blockson "began collecting at age 10, 'when no one was interested in black history.'" Blockson collected rare African American and African diaspora titles, with strong emphasis on Philadelphia and Pennsylvania, and the Underground Railroad. Among the rare material included in the collection are first editions of works by Phillis Wheatley, W. E. B. Du Bois, George Washington Williams, Paul Lawrence Dunbar, Johannes Capitein and Carter G. Williams. Blockson donated 20,000 books and pamphlets to Temple University in 1983. In 2006 he donated approximately ten thousand items, the majority of which were books, to the Penn State Library.[5]

John Henrik Clarke represents the second model, collecting for knowledge. Dr. Clarke allegedly read all or some portion of each book that he acquired, thus he is said to have collected for knowledge. Unlike Schomburg and Blockson, Clarke's focus was not on rare books and first editions. He himself mentions on more than one occasion that his universities were public libraries and well-stocked secondhand bookstores. The library would also have served a functional purpose as Dr. Clarke was the editor of *Freedomways*, a leading African American theoretical, political and cultural magazine (1961-1985). Clarke is thought to have had a personal library of more than 30,000 volumes in his home in Harlem. His basement library is said to often have been the locus for discussions and forums.[6]

Here Ard's schema may be tweaked a bit. Dr. Clarke actually straddles two of Ards' models. While he fits the collecting for knowledge category, he also fits the collecting for posterity model. Although his library is not comprised of rare books and first editions, it purports to be comprehensive in scope. It is an African diaspora collection of books focused primarily on African American history, religion, slavery, and literature (particularly that of Harlem Renaissance poets Langston Hughes and Countee Cullen), Africa and world history. The 20,000 volumes bequeathed to the Atlanta University Center is "noted for its material on blacks in the performing arts, race and apartheid, and includes every issue of *Presence Africaine*, the premier literary magazine of francophone Africa (1954 to 1985), of which Clarke was the most prolific English contributor."[7]

James Hatch and Camille Billops exemplify the collecting for empowerment model. The empowerment which their personal library bestows is its capacity to generate income and achieve a degree of financial success. Much of the collection's financial success came from Hatch's access to grants such as that from the National Endowment for the Humanities to conduct oral histories. The Hatch-Billops collection, built by theater historian James Hatch and artist and filmmaker Camille Billops, is limited in scope. Its subject focus is literature, music, theater, and the arts. The collection contains the complete works of of poet and dramatist Owen Dodson, original photographs of James VanDerZee, personal correspondence of playwright and director George C. Wolfe, oral histories with black artists, and so on. Since 1981 Hatch and Billops have published *Artist and Influence*, an annual that features transcripts of interviews, panel discussions, and forums. The Hatch-Billops collection was donated to the Manuscript, Archives, and Rare Book Library at Emory University in 2002.[8]

The fourth model in Ard's schema of black bibliophiles is "collecting for joy." Typifying this model is Portia Thompson, a federal employee, who maintains an informal community library in her home. One of its functions is to enable neighborhood children to complete their research projects, especially during Black History Month. Thompson contends that her greatest joy is passing on knowledge to the children so that her "investment in the collection will not go to waste." The collection of 2,000 books is of a size one would expect; such libraries vary widely from few items up to thousands. For instance, the personal library of clarinetist and college educator Michael White, containing nearly 4,000 books on jazz music, occupied five rooms of his home.[9]

In effect both Portia Thompson's and Michael White's personal libraries are working libraries. They have narrow subject scopes, plus they have specific functions. Michael White's collection of jazz books is typical of the personal working libraries associated with academics. As mentioned earlier, the usefulness of such libraries is the convenience of having resource material near at hand. Scope and specificity of function are inherent limitations of Portia Thompson's library as well. Her personal library functions both as a personal resource for herself and as a neighborhood resource for children. Ard's "collecting for joy" designation simply buries the idea that black personal libraries also can be *functional* working libraries.

Do Digital Collections Affect Black Bibliophiles?

The number of books published before Black Studies programs began in the late 1960s is relatively small. The sheer number of titles published now would make collecting comprehensively a daunting task. According to Valerie Sandoval Mwalino, "Early black collectors often attempted to document the total black experience in print, an ambitious goal, even in the nineteenth century. Today, one would require at least a ten-story building to house such a collection. Just to put things in perspective, the Schomburg Center spends over $100,000 every year acquiring books on black culture and we are by no means completely exhaustive in our holdings, even though we probably have 90 percent of what's available."[10] On the other hand, much of the allure of early black bibliophiles was their discovery and acquisition of hard-to-find rare books and or hitherto unknown titles by black authors. Today, or in the not too distant future, many of these kinds of book will probably be available in large digital collections.

In an essay on historical bibliography Abdul Alkalimat considers the transition from large personally amassed black heritage collections to digital collections. He cautions about the Google Books project: "A critical concern is what will be the impact of mainly digitizing books from the nineteenth century and before. We know that "racist false knowledge" was normative in the mainstream, so unless there is an active effort to digitize African American special collections the refutation of this misinformation will be absent, hence more legitimacy for racism. This is a serious concern for information professionals, as the resurrection of an immoral and unscientific past will do more harm than good." Randal Burkett has also spoken to this point, commenting that:

> White America, through institutions ranging from its leading universities to the Ku Klux Klan, began promulgating new notions of the inferiority of African Americans, predicated on spurious science and imagined history. As this new assault on black capabilities took form, a broad range of African American leadership from the worlds of politics, religion, cultural, and academic life recognized that they had to counter these falsehoods with their own accounts of their history.[11]

A narrow reading of Alkalimat leaves one with an impression that copies of books held by existing African American special collections are not in the Google Books or HathiTrust digital corpuses. Google Books is a combination of two digital book programs: the Library Project involves the scanning of books from major research libraries, while the Partners Program involves displaying materials provided by book publishers and rights holders. The latter allows for limited previews (snippets) of books still in copyright. Preservation projects such as Google Books and the HathiTrust Digital Library include tens of millions of digitized books scanned in cooperation with several major research libraries. Most books in these collections are in the public domain. Some were never copyrighted or the initial copyright not renewed, while others are "orphan works" for which no rights holder can be found.[12]

It is probably safe to surmise that Google and HathiTrust have digital copies of many of the books housed in African American special collections. So, shifting ground, the problem is not so much that Google or HathiTrust excludes the kinds of book collected by African American special collections, but that such books are undetectable within the two systems. Both Google's and HathiTrust's databases permit traditional subject searches and text mining to analyze texts about African Americans. However, both databases fall short of the level of adequacy desired by Alkalimat. One can search and/or analyze text data across millions of full-text documents in the two collections. The problem with search results about African Americans is that they are largely indiscriminate and fail to distinguish between racist and objective works of fact. Extending Alkalimat's line of reasoning, an "active effort to digitize African American special collections" might first start with coding bibliographic records. Subject descriptors or metadata tags that associate particular books with one or more African American special collections would help to alleviate the problem.

What links iconic black bibliophiles to the idealized digital corpus that Alkalimat imagines? In an ideal world African American digital collections are analogous to the personal libraries of black bibliophiles. The two themes, disseminating accurate information and building digital libraries comparable to black personal libraries, are implicit in a coauthored article by Abdul Alkalimat and Ron Bailey. They write: "Our mission is to guide and promote the journey of Black people into cyberspace … [by] digitizing our information, moving it from paper into digital files [and] …organizing these digital files into public use databases. These two tasks in the digital era take up the tasks initiated by W. E. B. Du Bois, Carter G. Woodson, Monroe Work, A. A. Schomburg, and many others in the twentieth century." The themes echo one voice decades earlier by James Turner, who also thought that scholars and bibliophiles should plan to preserve black collections with "our own resources, falling back on that which the black bibliophiles always had to rely on, community support." The sole difference being that in 1983 the medium of choice for preservation and wide-scale access was microfilm.[13]

As the Angela Ard schema reveals, there are several kinds of black bibliophile and collecting models. The two types represented by John Henrik Clarke and Portia Thompson are based on collecting for knowledge and personal growth. In addition, the Michael White jazz library was added to the conversation to make it clear that a fifth model should be added to the Ard schema, that black personal libraries can also be functional working libraries. Libraries of the latter type are the object of this study. Such personal libraries are aptly described by one book collector, who says: "I certainly like to think I know all of the books I have acquired… Even more important to me is my firm belief that I know what is inside of these volumes *on those occasions when I need to have the information they contain immediately at hand, which is the raison d'etre, after all, of a working library*" (italics mine, TW).[14]

Notes

1. Sinnette, Elinor Des Verney. (1990) "Arthur Alfonso Schomburg (1874-1938), Black Bibliophile and Collector." In Sinnette, Elinor Des Verney, W. Paul Coates, and Thomas C. Battle, eds. *Black Bibliophiles and Collectors: Preservers of Black History*. Washington, DC: Howard University Press, p. 35.

2. Hanes Walton, Jr. *Black Republicans: The Politics of the Black and Tan*. Metuchen, NJ: Scarecrow Press, 1975, p. iii; see also Walton, Hanes Jr. "The Literary Works of a Black Bibliophile: Clarence L. Holte," *Negro Educational Review* 29 (July/October 1978), p. 286. See also Britton, Helen H. "Dorothy Porter Wesley: Bibliographer, Curator, and Scholar." In Hildenbrand, Suzanne, ed. *Reclaiming the American Library Past*. Norwood, NJ: Ablex Publishing, 1996, p. 165; and Battle, Thomas C. "Moorland-Spingarn Research Center, Howard University." *Library Quarterly* 1988, 58(2), p. 143.

3. Brown, Allen. "Rules for Making the Most of Your Personal Library." *College English* 22, 1 (October 1960), p. 38 and 37. Otness, H. M. "A Room Full of Books: The Life and Slow Death of the American Residential Library." *Libraries and Culture*, 23, 2 (April 1988). Lee, Hur-Li. "The Concept of Collection from the User's Perspective." *Library Quarterly* 75, 1 (January 2005): 79.

4. Smith, Jessie Carney. *Black Academic Libraries and Research Collections: An Historical Survey*. Westport, CT: Greenwood Press, 1977, p.166. Also see Crowder, Ralph L. *John Edward Bruce: Politician, Journalist, and Self-trained Historian of the African diaspora*. New York: New York University Press, 2004, p. 119.

5. Sinnette, Elinor Des Verney Sinnette. *Arthur Alfonso Schomburg, Black Bibliophile and Collector*. Detroit: New York Public Library and Wayne State University Press, 1989. Blockson is discussed Angela Ards' "Professional and Amateur Collectors Indulge a Passion for Black History and Culture," *The Black Book Review*, February 28, 1996, p. 1.

6. Turner, James. "Summary." In Sinnette, Elinor Des Verney, W. Paul Coates and Thomas C. Battle, eds. *Black Bibliophiles and Collectors: Preservers of Black History*. Washington, DC: Howard University Press, 1990, p. 197.

7. Ards, Angela. "Professional and Amateur Collectors Indulge a Passion for Black History and Culture." *The Black Book Review*, February 28, 1996.

8. Ibid.

9. Ibid., p. 2; and "Straight Answers from Michael White," *American Libraries*, June-July, 2006, p. 26.

10. Mwalino, Valerie Sandoval. "The Arrangement and Care of Small Book Collections." In Elinor Des Verney Sinnette, W. Paul Coates and Thomas C. Battle, eds. *Black Bibliophiles and Collectors: Preservers of Black History*. Washington, DC: Howard University Press, 1990, p. 188.

11. Alkalimat, Abdul. "African American Bibliography: The social construction of a literature of record," November 2012, unpublished manuscript, p. 17; and Burkett, Randall. *The Mind of Carter G. Woodson*, p. 14.

12. Wilkin, John P. "Bibliographic Indeterminacy and the Scale of Problems and Opportunities of 'Rights' in Digital Collection Building," *Ruminations*, February 2011, http://www.clir.org/pubs/ruminations/index.html/01wilkin/wilkin.html.

13. Alkalimat, Abdul and Ronald Bailey. "From Black to eBlack: The Digital Transformation of Black Studies Pedagogy." *Fire!!!: The Multimedia Journal of Black Studies*, vol. 1, no. 1, p. 21. Alkalimat, Abdul. "African American Bibliography," p. 20. Turner, James. "Summary." In Elinor Des Verney Sinnette, W. Paul Coates and Thomas C. Battle, eds. *Black Bibliophiles and Collectors: Preservers of Black History* (Washington, DC: Howard University Press, 1990, p. 199].

14. Basbanes, Nicholas A. "Reflections on Personal Libraries." *Logos* 17, 1 (2006): 37-41.

CHAPTER TWO

Stances on Race Equality

Racial ideology is an organizing principle of black personal libraries. All three libraries, Ben Burns', Era Bell Thompson's, and Tom Dent's feature books on race relations and racial equality. Although each bibliophile believes in racial integration, their views on race identity and equality are not the same. For Ben Burns, integration means complete assimilation. This ranges from assimilation through race mixture and miscegenation to all aspects of social life. Era Bell Thompson emphasizes multiculturalism and equal opportunity in social areas. While civil rights and social integration are important for Tom Dent, he also endorses black cultural nationalism. For Dent, black identity should be defined in terms of black folk culture and African traditions rather than Western values. The differences between the three bibliophiles on identity and race equality are outlined further in ensuing paragraphs. Chapter 4 analyzes the way these differences are manifested in the individual collections.

Ben Burns

Ben Burns (Benjamin Bernstein, 1913-2000) graduated from the Northwestern University journalism program in 1934, joined the Communist Party a year later largely because of its social positions, and went on to ply his craft at three Communist newspapers, the *Daily Worker* (1937), *Midwest Daily Record* (1938), and the *People's World* (1940). Grounded in Communist social thought and advocacy journalism, he found employment at as a temporary editor at the *Chicago Defender* in 1942. There he assisted with the newspapers' two-part, 68-page supplement,"Victory Through Unity" to inspire African American support for the war effort. Burns himself authored an article in the supplement on employment dis-

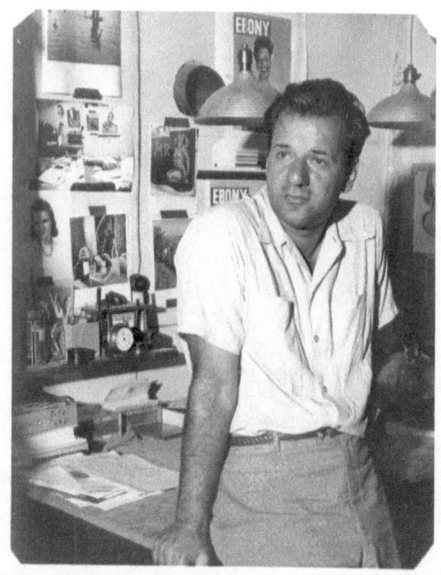

"Ben Burns in his office at Ebony, 1940s."
Credit to the Vivian Harsh Research Collection of Afro-American
History and Literature Collection, Chicago Public Library

crimination entitled "Let My People Work." Subsequently he would become the national editor of the *Chicago Defender* (1942-1946) and editor of the *Chicago Daily Defender* (1966-1967).[1]

An editor of the black press from 1943 to 1978, Ben Burns pioneered the first commercially successful African American magazine. As executive editor of the Johnson Publishing Company, he established a host of periodicals: the *Negro Digest* (1942-1954), *Ebony* (1945-1954), *Jet* (1950-1954), and *Tan Confessions* (founded 1950). After dismissal from the Johnson Publishing Company, he returned to public relations and became an executive in his own firm. Nestled between public relations work were several new editorial ventures, each relatively relatively short-lived. Only two issues of *Duke* (1957), a black magazine styled after *Playboy* magazine, were ever published. From 1956 to 1958 he also edited *Sepia*, a black magazine that rivaled *Ebony*. Burns' second turn at editing *Sepia* lasted from 1968 to 1977.

Identity and Race Equality

Socially and politically Burns was an avowed liberal. He proudly associates himself with various progressives and liberals that he worked with while at the *Chicago Defender*. In his autobiography he mentions routinely editing the columns of W. E. B. Du Bois, Langston Hughes, and Walter White, the secretary of the National Association for the Advancement of Colored People (NAACP). While Walter White was at best a liberal, Du Bois was a socialist and Hughes a communist. Burns' point is that because they shared similar views, the amount of editorial advice he needed to give was minimal.[2]

The themes of race mixture, interracial dating, miscegenation dominate Burns' social thought. Lilla van Saher's presentation copy of *Macamba* (1949), which is about biracial people, is inscribed "To Ben Burns who feels, writes works for the same ideals that I do!" Burns was not on the fringe with this way of thinking about race. Black community leaders as divergent as labor leader A. Philip Randolph and historian Carter G. Woodson endorsed this way of thinking. Insisting that the New Negro movement stands for unequivocal social equality, Randolph remarks "With respect to intermarriage, he maintains that it is the only logical, sound and correct aim for the Negro to entertain. He realizes that the acceptance of laws against intermarriage is tantamount to the acceptance of the stigma of inferiority." Woodson criticizes Charles S. Johnson's lack of courage to report that "the best evidence of recent improvement in race relations in the United States is the gradually increasing number of self-respecting and intelligent whites who are intermarrying with self-respecting and intelligent Negroes." [3]

The readers of *Jet* and *Ebony* magazines were enthralled by news of the interracial marriages of notables such as Pearl Bailey, Dorothy Dandridge, Lena Horne, Eartha Kitt, Richard Wright, and Walter White. Bailey, Dandridge, Horne, and Kitt were entertainers, Wright a renown literary author, and White a leader of the most powerful civil rights organization in the country. These relationships were offered as proof that whites could accept blacks as their social equals.[4] While advantageous to the Johnson Publishing Company at the time, in later years such stories would be regarded as sensationalist. The underlying racial ideology supporting it would be deposed as well.

It was in this context that an *Ebony* magazine staff meeting boiled over with agitation regarding a photograph of a black soldier kissing a white British woman. Burns sums up the issue between Era Bell Thompson and himself in the following terms:

> "It's just the kind of thing white folks always think Negro men dream about—to have a white woman. I know it'll get us circulation but I don't like it," Era Bell said sullenly. …She was a formidable antagonist in any wrangling over articles concerning sex or interracial romance, and we crossed swords frequently. … With my devout belief in total integration in every facet of everyday living, I was the recurrent spoiler in our repeated policy discord over racial mixing themes.[5]

While earlier issues of *Ebony* had capitalized on photo-journalism that featured interracial dating and marriage, Burns' continued emphasis of the theme had clearly fallen out of favor. Thus, John H. Johnson's termination letter pinpointed an apparently irreconcilable difference. He writes:

> In talking with you I've gotten the feeling that you are not personally aware of changes in thoughts and attitudes which have been going on in the Negro community and in the country as a whole. The over emphasis on sex, mixed marriage and other similar stories, which characterized and sparked our early growth and that of other publications, are no longer popular. Burns himself thought there was probably more to the matter than Johnson had said. Unwilling to believe he was terminated because of his racial ideology, he surmised the termination was due to his earlier Communist Party ties, or because *Ebony* was under criticism for having a white editor.[6]

Corroborating Burns' belief that there were other reasons for his termination, Era Bell Thompson refers to an attitudinal problem. Apparently, Burns relations with coworkers left much to be desired. According to Thompson:

> We had a white supervisor at one time who just didn't like people. If they were black, that made it worse. Mr. Johnson told us that as soon as Herbert Nipson and I were able to take over, he

would get rid of this guy. I thought it would never happen, but it did. First he wanted to be sure that we knew how to run the magazine before he put it in our hands.[7]

Believing that his Communist Party affiliation or, because the nation's premiere black magazine was run by a white man, may have been at the root of his problems, Burns seems to have been unaware that office relationships and morale were poor.

Era Bell Thompson

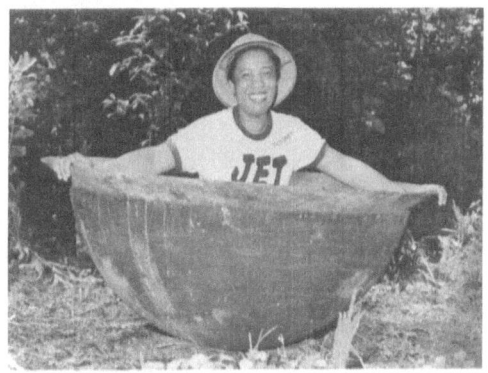

Source: State Historical Society of North Carolina

Era Bell Thompson, 1905-1986, was an autobiographer, prose writer, and editor. In the 1920s she published poetry and prose for the *Chicago Defender* under the pseudonym Dakato Dick. In 1947 John H. Johnson hired her as managing editor of his magazine *Negro Digest*, later retitled *Black World* under the editorship of Hoyt Fuller. Years later (1954) Thompson was appointed as one of two associate editors of *Ebony* and named Johnson Publishing Company's International Editor in 1964. She wrote numerous editorials, the *Negro Digest* editorial column was called "Bell's Lettres," and more than forty feature articles for *Ebony*. Era Bell Thompson also authored two books (*American Daughter* in 1946 and *Africa Land of My Fathers* in 1954). The books were overshadowed by similar books published around the same time by Richard Wright (*Black Boy*, 1945; and *Black Power: A Record of Reactions in a Land of Pathos*, 1954).[8]

Identity and Race Equality

The ideas of race and equal opportunity are bound together in Era Bell Thompson's thinking about multiculturalism. Her biographer notes that "Integration for Thompson does not mean assimilation—losing one's black identity by merging completely with the surrounding white world—but involves rather a mixing of cultural elements, as symbolized in one example by her brothers developing their own patois, which they dub "Negrowegian." Elsewhere, Thompson herself speaks about equal opportunity and race equality: "I found that if you excel, if you can outdo the other fellow, well, usually they'll accept you. But you have to prove it, you have to forever be proving something." [9]

In part, Thompson's thinking about race equality is fashioned from witnessing her father's mastery over an assortment of occupations in various locales throughout the Midwest. Stewart Caval Thompson, an ex-slave, was both a self-determined and industrious individual. Moving from place to place he took advantage of the opportunities available to him. He was a farmer, coal miner, labor union treasurer, assistant at both the Iowa state Senate and North Dakota Senate, a private messenger to North Dakota Governor Lynn J. Frazier, a restaurant chef, and finally, as owner of a second-hand furniture store. Also, a racial model gaining traction in the 1940s was that racial prejudice could be controlled by attacking discrimination which denies equal access to the opportunity.[10]

Thompson's multiculturalism and racial tolerance stems from her Midwestern upbringing. She belonged to the only black family in Driskoll, North Dakota and was one of the few blacks to attend area schools and colleges. Furthering her sense of multiculturalism was Dr. Richard Riley, a white Methodist minister from North Dakota, and his family. Shortly after her father passed away, Thompson became all but a member of the Riley family, living with Dr. Riley, his wife Susan, their son Jan, and Dr. Riley's younger brother Glen.

In exchange for helping with the house work, Riley offered her an opportunity to resume her college education at the University of Dakota. The Women's Guild of his church provided a scholarship to cover tuition and books. She transferred to Morningside College, a Methodist school in Iowa, when Dr. Riley became its president. Taken altogether, these things made her "less prejudiced against whites than the average black." In an interview Thompson says "There are quite a lot of things that I don't believe in, such as differences in people." [11]

Ellen DeFreece-Wilson believes Thompson's multiculturalism was also influenced by the W. E. B. DuBois' novel, *Dark Princess: A Romance* (1928). Supposedly this was Thompson's favorite book. This is an important, although somewhat understated, point. Reading the Du Bois novel pinpoints a moment in the late-1920s when Thompson's multiculturalism expands to include race pride as well. While tolerant of other cultures, pride in her own race was absent in her self-understanding. In her own words, "*The Dark Princess* impressed me more than did any of the others, for never before had I heard black beautified, Negroes exalted." With the revelation of the Du Bois novel came awareness of Harlem Renaissance writers, Claude McKay, Langston Hughes, Rudolph Fisher, and others.

Continuing along this trajectory, some 15 of so years later Thompson takes a job at *Ebony* to learn more about her people, work which "made her think black for the first time." [12]

Tom Dent

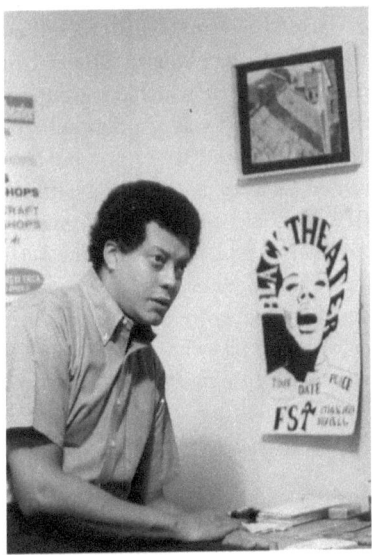

A photograph of Tom Dent pictured with a poster of the Free Southern Theater. Copyrighted by the Amistad Research Center.

Tom Dent (Thomas Covington Dent, 1932-1998) was a journalist, poet, playwright, prose writer, cultural institution builder, and editor of the black press. In the 1950s Dent was a reporter for the *Houston Informer* and the *New York Age*, both black weekly newspapers. Between 1961 and 1963 he was the public relations officer for the National Association for the Advancement of Colored People Legal Defense Fund. There he worked under Thurgood Marshall for several months before the latter was appointed to the United States Court of Appeals for the Second Circuit. Thereafter Dent worked with attorneys Jack Greenberg and Constance Baker Motley. Thurgood Marshall would later become an Associate Justice of the United States Supreme Court (1967-1991), Jack Greenberg became the Director-Counsel of the NAACP Legal Defense Fund (1961-1984), and Constance Baker Motley became federal judge for the Southern District of New York (1966-1986).

Among Tom Dent's credits as an institution builder, he co-founded the *Umbra* workshop, a collective of young black writers based in Manhattan's Lower East Side. He was also the editor of the group's literary magazine *Umbra*. Dent founded BlackArtsSouth, a writer's group affiliated with the Free Southern Theater. He edited their literary magazine, *Nkombo*. Later he founded the Congo Square Writers' Union and was editor of the one-issue *Black River Journal* which the group sponsored. Another organization that he co-founded was the Southern Black Cultural Alliance, a federation of community theater groups. Lastly, he co-founded a literary journal named *Callaloo*, co-editing the first couple of issues.[13]

Dent authored two books of poetry, *Magnolia Street* (1976) and *Blue Lights and River Songs* (1982). Under contract (1984-1986) to assist with Andrew Young's autobiography, a childhood friend and long-time associate, Dent researched and wrote earlier drafts. Eventually the editor brought in another writer to take the narrative in a different direction. The end product was titled *An Easy Burden* (1996). Based on interviews collected in 1991, he authored his third book *Southern Journey* (1997) which revisits places where protesters took a stand for equality.[14]

Identity and Race Equality

As a Black Arts Movement poet and cultural activist Tom Dent was concerned with black consciousness and identity formation. For young writers such as Dent during the post-Civil Rights Movement period, black cultural nationalism replaced the ideal of race equality through integration. Dent expresses this in one of his letters, writing "The black man ... stands in critical posture to the culture & beliefs of western European civilization—he has every right to exist in his fullest powers whether western european culture has a *place* for him or not."[15] The idea of basing black identity and race equality on the approval by whites is replaced by normative standards based on black life and culture.

An example of the shifting terrain for authenticity and value judgements concerns the mixed reception given William Styron's Pulitzer Prize winning novel *The Confessions of Nat Turner* (1967). Commenting about Styron's portrayal of Nat Turner and the Virginia slave rebellion, Dent says:

> It's the wildest thing. Such a violent polarity between what the black cats are saying and what the white literary establishment is saying. ...I mean there's just no meeting ground anywhere between what these people are saying. ...[You] must read the review of *Eight Black Writers Respond*, or something like that, by a white historian, Genovese. I sort of tend to agree with him, at least...that we have to write our own interpretations, either as history or fiction, of our heroes if we don't like what white writers do.[16]

While lauded by "the white literary establishment," Styron's novel drew criticism from black intellectuals. Dent thinks black writers have a responsibility to critique negative portrayals and correct misinterpretations about black culture. Moreover, he thinks that the justifications for judgements about black identity and self-worth are found in black cultural traditions. He says as much in a letter to fellow poet, Alvin Aubert. Dent writes:

> I think the image of the ideal *sharing* black brother or sister is what keeps me from writing down to black people (and keeps me searching through our writings even in unlikely places), for no matter how presently worthless American society may consider our efforts we are the guardians of certain hidden truths, secret stories the real stories of the journeys of our people.[17]

Together with Calvin Hernton, David Henderson, Joe Johnson, Roland Snellings (Askia M. Toure) and Brenda Walcott, Dent founded the Umbra writers workshop in 1962. Other young writers belonging to the collective, with whom Dent corresponded long after his Lower East Side Manhattan days with Umbra, were LeRoi Jones (Imamu Amiri Baraka), Ishmael Reed, and James Thompson. Umbra was considered to be at the center of the Black Arts Movement. It provided a forum for poets to perform their compositions and published an important black literary magazine. First published in March, 1963, the *Umbra* magazine contributed to redirecting black racial ideology from its focus from cultural integration to the critique of Western values.[18]

Returning home to New Orleans, Dent became the associate director of the Free Southern Theater. The Free Southern Theater, a cultural project loosely allied with the civil rights oriented Student Nonviolent Coordinating Committee, was one of the more cohesive of the Black Arts Movement's drama collectives. Dent proposes a recalibrated vision for the Free Southern Theater, writing that:

> The value of the FST as I see it has to do with psychology, with an attack on the racist psychology of the United States, whether crass or genteel, and an attack on the self-denigrating psychology of Black communities, and especially, because this is where the potential lies, on the self-denigrating psychology of Black Youth. This attack can be philosophical through the shows, but it can also be through simple exposure to racial reality through history, discussion, and the availability of materials like books which are not now and never have been available to Black youth. The books which we used in the workshops last year are not available in the public schools or colleges. The discussions after shows and around the FST do not happen in any other social institution of the Black community. This is our importance and value.[19]

In addition, Dent went on to establish BlackArtsSouth (1968-1973) as a literary wing of the Free Southern Theater. This was the second of his three writers workshop. After breaking ties with the Free Southern Theater, he began a third group was named the Congo Square Writers' Union. About the third writers' group, he says "it was just a descendent of the writing workshop I had with the Free Southern Theater, which was a descendent of the Umbra workshop. But it was more than a writing workshop, obviously. It was a fellowship of people who had the same artistic yearnings, if not artistic production. It was a fellowship of friends."[20]

Notes

1. Burns, Ben. *Nitty Gritty: A White Editor in Black Journalism*. Jackson, MS: University Press of Mississippi, 1996, p. 5.

2. Burns, Ben. *Nitty Gritty*, p. 14.

3. Randolph, A. Philip. "The New Negro—What Is He?" *The Messenger* 2 (August 1920); and Carter G. Woodson. "Review of *Into the Main Stream, a Survey of Best Practices in Race Relations*." *Journal of Negro History*, July 1947, 32 (3): 372.

4. Romano, Renee. "Marriage, Mixed." In Finkelman, Paul, ed. *Encyclopedia of African American History 1896 to Present: From the Age of Segregation to the Twenty-First Century*. New York: Oxford University Press, 2009, p. 259.

5. Burns, Ben. *Nitty Gritty*, p. 139.

6. Ibid., p. 189, 190.

7. Thompson, Era Bell and Marcia M. Greenlee. *Interview with Era Bell Thompson, March 6 and 10, 1978*, p. 39; Burns, Ben. *Nitty Gritty*, p. 90.

8. DeFreece-Wilson, Eileen, "Era Bell Thompson," p. 25; p. 160.

9. Johnson, Michael K. "'This Strange White World': Race and Place in Era Bell Thompson's American Daughter." *Great Plains Quarterly* 24 (Spring 2004), p. 107; Thompson, Era Bell and Marcia M. Greenlee. *Interview with Era Bell Thompson, March 6 and 10, 1978*. Cambridge, MA: Schlesinger Library, Radcliffe College, p. 39, 41.

10. MacIver, Robert M. *The More Perfect Union: A Program for the Control of Inter-Group Discrimination in the United States*. New York: Macmillan, 1948, p. 126-127.

11. Thompson, Era Bell, *American Daughter*, pp. 216, 224, 230; and Thompson, Era Bell and Marcia M. Greenlee, *Interview with Era Bell Thompson*, pp. 39, 41.

12. DeFreece-Wilson, Eileen, "Era Bell Thompson," p. 163; Thompson, Era Bell, *American Daughter*, p. 178, 197; Ibid., pp. 38, 44; and Crimmins, Jerry. "Black editor, author Era Bell Thompson, 80." *Chicago Tribune*, December 31, 1986, section 2, p. 8.

13. Ward, Jerry W., Jr. "The Art of Tom Dent: Notes on Early Evidence." *African American Review* 40.2 (2006): 320; Thomas, Lorenzo. "The Need to Speak: Tom Dent and the Shaping of a Black Aesthetic." *African American Review* 40.2 (2006): 325; and Drake, Jennifer. "Dent, Tom." In Gates, Henry Louis Jr. and Evelyn Brooks Higginbotham, eds. *African American National Biography*. Oxford African American Studies Center, http://www.oxfordaasc.com/article/opr/t0001/e1393 (accessed March 8, 2012).

14. Ward, Jerry W. Jr. "Dent, Tom." In Andrews, William L., Frances Smith Foster and Trudier Harris, eds. *The Concise Oxford Companion to African American Literature*. Oxford African American Studies Center, http://www.oxfordaasc.com/article/opr/t52/e153 (accessed March 8, 2012).

15. Turner, Lorenzo. "The Need to Speak: Tom Dent and the Shaping of a Black Aesthetic," p. 333; Thomas, Lorenzo. "Tom Dent." In Thadious M. Davis and Trudier Harris, eds. *Afro-American Writers after 1955: Dramatists and Prose Writers*. Detroit: Gale Research Co., 1985, p. 90.

16. Thomas Covington Dent Papers, Amistad Research Center, Tulane University, New Orleans, Louisiana. Letter to David Henderson, Sept. 8, 1968. Thomas Covington Dent Papers. Series I: O.Correspondence, 1955-56, 1966-67. Box 24: Folder 2.

17. Thomas Covington Dent Papers, Amistad Research Center, Tulane University, New Orleans, Louisiana. Letter to Alvin Aubert. 12/23/77. O.Correspondence, 1977. Box 25: Folder 1.

18. Thomas, Lorenzo. "The Need to Speak: Tom Dent and the Shaping of a Black Aesthetic." *African American Review* 40.2 (2006): 327; Ibid., p. 330.

19. Thomas Covington Dent Papers, Amistad Research Center, Tulane University, New Orleans, Louisiana. Letter to Members of Board of Directors, General Manager, Company Manager. June 4, 1967. Correspondence, 1967. Box 1: Folder 10.

20. Ward, Jerry W. Jr. "Tom Dent talking: New Orleans as a resource of genius." *Xavier Review* 6.1 (1986): p. 2.

CHAPTER THREE

Experiences in Book Collecting: A Bibliographic Essay

It is a truism (or should be) that most books in an individual's personal library have been selected and/or purchased by that individual. Prima facie, a book's mere presence in a personal collection suggests it was acquired through purchase. On the other hand, while most books in a collection were probably purchased, few offer incontrovertible proof of this such as cancelled personal checks, sales receipts, markings from second-hand book dealers, publisher brochures or catalogs with marked selections, etc. For example, enclosed in one of Ben Burns' books (Benjamin Quarles' *Negro in the American Revolution*) is a sales receipt from Kroch's and Brentano's, one of the largest bookstores in Chicago. In addition to a trail of cancelled checks payable to bookstores and publishers, Tom Dent's correspondence has several makes reference to finding books at conferences. In his own words, "that's why I go." [1]

Ben Burns

Ben Burns was hired by the *Chicago Defender* when the newspaper needed extra writers to publish its legendary "Victory Through Unity" edition in September, 1942. From that first assignment, he claims to have began studying the black community almost like a sociologist, filling "file folders with tidbits of information about who-was-who in Chicago's Bronzeville and what organizations made the South Side neighborhood tick." Commenting further, Burns says:

> With the concentrated study of a Talmudic scholar, I endeavored in my early *Defender* days to learn as much as I could in the shortest possible time about Negro history and culture. I

soon discovered that I was more knowledgeable than many of my colleagues and encouraged the reporters to read more about black history as well as current racial events to broaden their knowledge of subjects that in those days were neglected in school curriculums.[2]

Associates at the *Chicago Defender* thought of him as a bibliophile "whose knowledge descends from a lifetime of study." In the same vein, referring to Burn's adjustment at the *Chicago Defender* and Johnson Publications, his daughter has said: "He was a very voracious reader. He studied everything." [3]

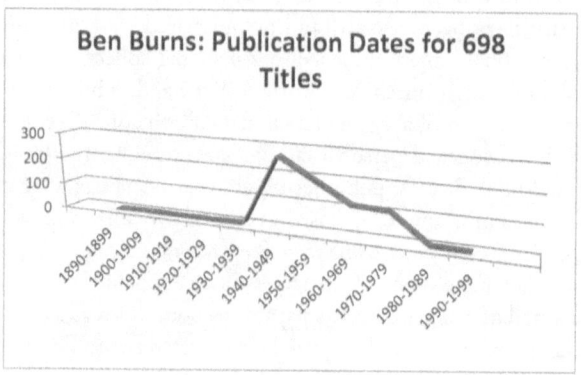

Figure 1: Publication Dates of Burns Collection Titles

Altogether 698 of the 755 books in the Ben Burns library are included in this study. The excluded titles are romance and mystery novels, books on journalism and broadcasting techniques, duplicate titles, various editions of a a title, and works that were not black-oriented or race-related. Figure 1 indicates that Burns' collecting activity peaked from the late 1930s to mid-1940s. The peak years correspond to his work as columnist and editor of the *Chicago Defender* national edition. While working for the *Defender* Burns edited *Negro Digest* and *Ebony* magazines, founded in 1943 and 1945, respectively. Possibly mistrustfulness, the idea that his loyalties were divided, led to his dismissal from the *Defender*.

Many of the books in Burns' personal library are retrospective acquisitions, i.e., published before he began his long tenure as an editor of the black press. There is a distinction between when a book is published and when it is purchased. However, because the magazine editors and book reviewers examined here were chiefly concerned with contemporary issues, the distinction is of small concern. There are 16 retrospective acquisitions in the Burns library. These include two 19th century books of poetry by Paul Laurence Dunbar and early 20th century works by Dunbar, Booker T. Washington, and W. E. B. Du Bois.

Dunbar's poetry includes *Poems of Cabin and Field* (1899), *Lyrics of Love and Laughter* (1903), book plated "Ex Libris From Edward J. Ward, no. 171, class poet, 30 Aug. 1904"; contains both sentimental and somberly realistic expressions and depictions of black life, and it features both dialect and standard English verse. *Lyrics of Lowly Life* (1896), inscribed "J. F. Nuner, Apr. 27, 1906"; and *Lyrics of Sunshine and Shadow* (1905), inscribed "To my husband - J. F. N. - Birthday Greetings. Apr. 27, 1906. RRBN." The other books published in this time period are Booker T. Washington's autobiography *Up from Slavery* (1907) and W. E. B. Du Bois' *The Negro* (1915), a history of African descended peoples from their early cultures through the slave trade and into the 20th century.

Books between 1929 and 1940 include Caldwell's *We are the living* (1933), a book of short stories about Southern culture which includes "Picking cotton" and "Yellow girl"; Langston Hughes' autobiography *The big sea* (1940) in which he discusses his life from 1902 up to 1930. Other books within the time period are Richard A. Loederer's *Voodoo fire in Haiti* (1935); Horace R. Cayton's *Black Workers and the New Unions* (1939); John George Van Deusen's *"Brown Bomber": The Story of Joe Louis* (1940); and Karl Marx and Frederick Engels' *Civil War in the United States* (1937).

A number of books found in the Burns library were accumulated in connection with his book reviewing activities. Of the 698 books in the collection, 144 are review copies. Evidence a book's status as a review copy are identifiable stamps, flyers, or publication release notices within the books, etc. Unfortunately, some flyers and release notices may have been removed, possibly resulting in an undercount of the real number of review books. When writing for Communist Party newspapers in the late 1930s Burns would keep the books that he reviewed. He continued the practice in the 1940s when he joined the *Chicago Defender*. He writes:

> When I became book reviewer for the *Defender*, I would take home up to a dozen books a week. Most of them were on ra-

cial subjects, and I poured over these books incessantly to learn more about the rich history of centuries of ceaseless Negro endeavor to win a measure of equality in America.[4]

John H. Johnson's first magazine was the *Negro Digest* (1942) and was modeled after a best-selling popular magazine, *Readers' Digest*. The latter condensed articles of topical interest and entertainment value from other periodicals. Remarking on the start up of *Negro Digest*, Burns notes that he "did all the editorial work and makeup of the first issue at home on my kitchen table, much of it after a long day of house painting in the morning and followed by hours of work at either the *Defender* or the Dickerson or Dawson campaign offices." [5]

Welcoming the publicity given their racial works, publishers would send books and advanced galley proofs to the magazine for possible use. "A notable coup," writes Burns, "was publication of a chapter from Lillian Smith's controversial novel *Strange Fruit*, before its publication date. Part of Richard Wright's *Black Boy* ran in *Negro Digest* before the book was pubished." *Strange Fruit* (1944) is a novel about the prelude and aftermath of a lynching in Georgia, depicting the South's racial problems. Burns' copy has his ownership inscription and is annotated. Richard Wright's *Black Boy* (1945) is an autobiographical novel that explores the author's early life in Mississippi. Burns has annotated it as well.[6]

While *Negro Digest* and *Ebony* are at the front end Burns' career as a magazine editor, at the end is his editorship of *Sepia*. *Sepia* magazine rivaled *Ebony* and was comparable in terms of photographic and journalistic content. A notable book added to Burns' personal library is Langston Hughes and Milton Meltzer's *A Pictorial History of the Negro in America* (1963). This is a pictorial work with biographical and historical material about African American life from pre-revolutionary times to the civil rights movement. Inserted in the book is a handwritten enclosure with directions from Burns about the layout of a review article with photographs in *Sepia*.

There are remarkably few gift books in Burns' library. In all there were only 23. There may be other gifts in the collection but, because they are unmarked, we have no way of knowing which books these are. Twelve of the 23 gift books are inscribed by their authors to Burns. Books published between 1942 and 1949 are Howard W. Coles' *The Cradle of Freedom: A History of the Negro in Rochester, Western New York and Canada*

(1942), a history of antislavery movements; Bucklin Moon's *Primer for White Folks* (1945), an anthology of prose writings by and about African Americans; and Eslanda Goode Robeson's *African Journey* (1945) which describes her trip to East and South Africa.

John Roeburt's novel *Seneca, U. S. A.* (1947) is about newspaper editor forced to comply with the conservative leanings of the paper's owner with regards to post-war unrest, labor unions, and race relations; Earl Conrad's *Jim Crow America* (1947), about economic conditions, rural-urban migration, housing segregation, etc.; Lilla van Saher's novel *Macamba* (1949) which deals with the identity crisis of a biracial, multi-religious (Jewish, Catholic), man who lives on a Caribbean island. The Southside Community Committee's *Bright Shadows in Bronzetown* (1949) is a history of their community work in Chicago black neighborhoods; and Langston Hughes' *One-Way Ticket* (1949) is a book of poetry.

Two gift books in Burns' personal library are inscribed to John H. Johnson, owner of the Johnson Publishing Company. These are Frederick Leslie Brownlee's *New day ascending* (1946) which is a short history of the American Missionary Association beginning in 1839 when a cargo of Africans mutinied aboard the Spanish schooner Amistad. The book has been annotated by Burns. The other book is Peter Noble's *Negro in films* (1949), an early book on the history of blacks in Hollywood and British films with chapters on actors, silent films, musicals, and post war films.

There are four gift books that were published between 1950 and 1973. A. S. Young's *Great Negro Baseball Stars, and How They Made the Major Leagues* (1953) tells how blacks broke through segregation into the major leagues and how they have been faring. Lerone Bennett's *Before the Mayflower; A History of the Negro in America, 1619-1962* (1962) traces black history from the great empires of western Africa to the civil rights upheavals of the 1960s and 1970s. Langston Hughes' *Something in Common, and Other Stories* (1963) is a collection of 37 short stories presenting a cross section of his work as a short-story writer; and Ruth Duckett Gibbs' *Black is the Color* (1973) is a book of poetry for juveniles that is illustrated by artist Tom Feelings.

The remaining books with inscriptions indicate prior ownership. These are inscribed to unknown individuals and/or have the imprints of book dealers, libraries, or schools. The three Dunbar poetry books mentioned earlier belong to this group. Ben Burns probably purchased the three poetry books from antiquarian book dealers or at auction. Because the other books are more recent, they may have been purchased from secondhand bookstores or library book sales. A reprint of Carter Godwin Woodson's classic *Mis-education of the Negro* (1969), originally published in 1933, focuses on the affect that cultural indoctrination has had on African Americans with regards to education, employment and social conditions. Evidently the book's route to Burns was a circuitous one. It appears to have first belonged to the Chicago school system as it is stamped "Board of Education, City of Chicago." Subsequently it was owned by an Eva S. Butler, as it bears her inscription.

Other books suggestive of prior ownership are Henri Ch. Rosemond's 12-scene play *Haiti: Our Neighbor* (1944), inscribed by Rosemond to someone other than Burns. Edwin Rozwenc's *Reconstruction in the South* (1952) is stamped "Beverly Paper-Back Exchange 239-0163." It is an anthology of essays about political reconstruction in southern states after the Civil War. Wilman Dykeman and Janes Stokely's *Neither Black Nor White* (1957) is inscribed by the authors to Reverend and Mrs. Berggren. This is a collection of interviews and conversations with black and white Southerners about segregation. Lorraine Hansberry's drama *A Raisin in the Sun* (1959) is inscribed by its previous owner M. Sager and is about housing segregation in Chicago. Comedian and activist Dick Gregory satirizes about segregation in *From the Back of the Bus* (1962). The book is inscribed "To Dave Hepburn with my very best wishes, Dick Gregory."

Era Bell Thompson

In his critique of a book about black bibliophiles, Donald Franklin Joyce draws attention to its weak coverage of bibliophiles from the non-Eastern United States. Among the Midwestern bibliophiles he thinks are deserving of attention is Era Bell Thompson.[7] Altogether 362 of a total 394 books are included in this study. Books that were omitted cover an assortment of health books and books about the fields of journalism and communications.

Figure 2 shows an uptick in Era Bell Thompson's collecting activity from the late-1930s to late-1950s, peaking during the late-1950s and 1960s. The first period corresponds with her work as a copy editor for the *Chicago Defender*, the publishing of her autobiography *American Daughter* (1946), and her recruitment by John H. Johnson to become editor of

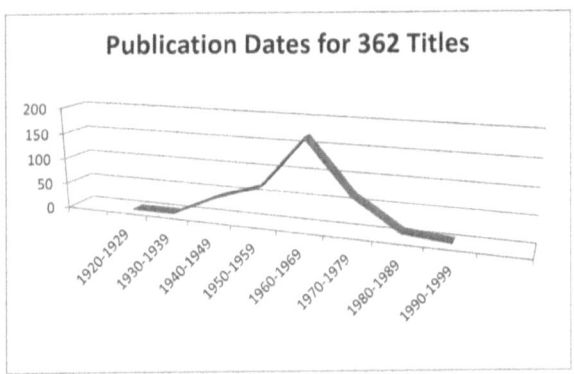

Figure 2: Publication Dates of Thompson Collection Titles

the *Negro Digest* (1947) and associate editor of *Ebony* (1947-1951). Her peak collecting period coincides with the ten-year period in which she was managing co-editor of *Ebony* (1951-1964), published her second autobiography *Africa: Land of My Fathers* (1954), co-edited *White on Black* (1963), an anthology of essays written by whites reflecting their views about blacks, and became the Johnson Publishing Company's international editor (1964-1986).

The retrospect acquisitions in Thompson's library include all books published before 1947, when she became editor of the *Negro Digest*. Several books from this period were supplemental to her writing *American Daughter*. These include Bruce Opie Nelson's *Land of the Dacotahs* (1946), a history of Native Americans in the Northwest; and Lloyd Wendt's *Bright Tomorrow* (1945), a novel set in the Midwest farming country about a young man whose German background and individualistic father stop him from integrating into the community. Also within this group are the London and Chicago imprints of *American Daughter* (1946) published by Victor Gollancz and the University of Chicago Press, respectively. Other older books may have served as research or background material for her *Negro Digest* and *Ebony* magazine articles. These include E. Allen and C. C. Lacaita's travel guide *Ravello* (1926), a picturesque coastal town in southern Italy known to have inspired several authors and artists; Donald Pierson's *Negroes in Brazil, a Study of Race Contact at Bahia* (1942), about the social conditions of black Brazilians; Emily Post's *Etiquette: The Blue Book of Social Usage* (1945); and *Roget's*

International Thesaurus (1946).

Thompson's *Negro Digest* columns were titled "Bell's Lettres" (1949-1951). The early columns dealt with her travels throughout the South even though she "knew nothing about black people, the South, or any of the racial situations common to black existence in the southern states." [8] Several retrospective titles about black life in the region would have alleviated this deficiency. J. Saunders Redding's *No day of triumph* (1942) describes his automobile trip through black America to see how people lived in the South. The Federal Writers' Project's *These Are Our Lives* (1939) is a collection of narratives about the South from former slaves. Benjamin Albert Botkin's *Lay My Burden* (1945) describes white and black southerners. Hurston's *Dust Tracks on a Road* (1942) is an account of childhood poverty in the rural South; and Lillian Smith's *Strange Fruit* (1944) is a novel about race relations in the South before and after a lynching.

A portion of Thompson's personal library is due to her book reviewing activities. Generally these are marked by a flyer, a publisher's announcement or review notice, or were was reviewed in the "Books," or "Book of the Week" sections of *Jet* magazine. Longer reviews in *Jet* often ended with the initials "EBT." Quite possibly many more books are more review copies, but the identifying insignia have been removed. Thompson suggests that her interest reviewing books began in the 1920s while working several months for one of Chicago's black magazines. Writing about the experience, she says "For the first time I read books written by Negroes, and when Mr. Moore learned of my interest in writing I earned an extra dollar for each book I reviewed." Except for the E. Allen and C. C. Lacaita travel guide mentioned earlier, no other book in her library was published in the 1920s. In particular W. E. B. DuBois' *The Dark Prince*, mentioned as one of her favorite novels, is not in her book collection.[9]

In addition to reviewing books for Johnson Publishing Company magazines, Thompson did reviews for other national media. Among these are the *BMI Book Parade* (Broadcast Music, Inc.), *Chicago Sun-Times*, *Chicago Tribune*, and the *New York Herald Tribune*. Her review essay of books about blacks for the young reader is featured in "The Junior Bookshelf," *Chicago Sun-Times* (January 2, 1966). A pair of books reviewed in the *Chicago Sun-Times* are suggestive of Thompson's racial ideology. Jesse Owens' *Blackthink: My Life as a Black Man and White Man*

(1970) opines that Black Power radicals benefited greatly from the civil rights movement of the 1950s and 1960s and that their ongoing agitation was unfounded. Thompson has annotated this book. Leslie Alexander Lacy's autobiography *The Rise and Fall of a Proper Negro* (1970) tracks a shift in racial ideology, from the desire to emulate and integrate to the need to separate and achieve identity. A copy of this book is not in the Thompson library.

Another review essay in the *Chicago Sun-Times* is "Four Books put Africa into New Proper Focus." The four books under consideration are John C. Caldwell and Elsie F. Caldwell's *Our Neighbors in Africa* (1961), a brief introduction with timely topics including modern war problems, a glimpse at big cities, and Albert Schweitzer; Maud A. Barker-Benfield's *The Lands and Peoples of East Africa* (1961), a geography textbook for young adults aged fifteen to sixteen; Sam Olden's *Getting to Know Africa's French Community* (1960), a travel piece highlighting 12 newly independent states, including a section about the many ways in which Africa has benefited from France; and Katharine Savage's *The Story of Africa: South of the Sahara* (1961). Several Thompson book reviews were recorded radio programs and aired nationally. Continuity from Broadcast Music, Inc. recorded and transcribed her reviews of Willa Cather's *My Antonia* (1954); Majorie Kinnan Rawlings' *The Sojourner* (1955); *Truman Capote's The Muses are Heard* (1957); and George W. Shepherd, Jr.'s *They Wait in Darkness*. This entire group of books is absent from Thompson's library.[10]

In light of Thompson's stellar reputation as a book reviewer, Langston Hughes and Arna Bontemps extended her an invitation to serve on the Advisory Board of their Negro Book Society. In his letter to Thompson, Hughes writes: "Tentatively, our plans call for the selection of four books per year, and as a Board member we would like you to participate in the quarterly selection." Believing that serving both the Negro Book Society and Johnson Publishing might be a conflict of interest, she was obliged to decline the offer.[11]

Two of Thompson's primary interests are religion and racial ideology. Both were fostered by an association with Methodist minister Dr. Richard Riley and his family. Riley was "hepped up about Negroes and education," helping both Thompson and her friend Muriel return to college with the assistance of the Women's Guild of his church. Also, family life with the Riley's complemented the early multiracialism she had learned during her formative years in North Dakota. Of the several religious books in Thompson's personal library, three are bibles. These are *Good News for Modern Man: The New Testament in Today's English Version* (1966); the *Good News Bible: The Bible in Today's English Version* (1976); and the *Holy Bible: Old & New Testaments: King James Version: Translated Out of the Original Tongues and with Previous Translations Diligently Compared and Revised: Presented Side by Side with the Living Bible, Paraphrased, a Thought-for-Thought Translation* (1981).

Other religious books have a more or less proselytizing nature. These are *New African Saints: The Twenty-Two Martyrs of Uganda* (1964), an account of the Ugandan Christians who were murdered for their written especially for youth, with many color illustrations. William. J. Lederer's *Timothy's Song* (1965) about a hunchbacked newspaper boy at the turn of the 19th century who leads a life of loneliness, hardship, and tragedy, but is rewarded after his death by God in heaven. The book is inscribed by the author to Thompson. Robert L. Short's *The Parables of Peanuts* (1968) delivers certain religious themes selected from the *Peanuts* newspaper comic strips of Charles M. Schulz.

Other books cover missionaries, the black church, and non-Christian religions. Books about African missionaries include James H. Robinson's *Road without Turning* (1950), an autobiography of the Presbyterian minister who founded *Operation Crossroads Africa*, a cross-cultural exchange program and forerunner of the *Peace Corps*. Basil Davidson's *The African Awakening* (1955), an account of the underlying reasons for the current troubles of Africa; Charlotte Crogman Wright's *Beneath the Southern Cross: The Story of an American Bishop's Wife in South Africa* (1955); and Oma Lou Myers' *Rosa's Song: The Life and Ministry of Rosa Page Welch* (1984). Welch, a famed gospel singer and missionary, was heralded as the "Ambassador of Goodwill" for her efforts to better interracial relations. The book is inscribed to Thompson by the author.

E. Franklin Frazier's *The Negro Church in America* (1964) begins with an analysis of how Christianity provided slaves with a basis for social cohesion and ends with the black church's diminishing importance as increasing numbers of blacks become urbanized and integrated into the American mainstream. Leonidas H. Berry's *I Wouldn't Take Nothin' for My Journey* (1981) chronicles the impact of the African Methodist Episcopal Church on the lives of several generations of his family. The book is inscribed by the author to Thompson.

E. Bolaji Idowu' *African Traditional Religion: A Definition* (1973) objects to a long history of derogatory evaluations of Africans and their culture by outsiders. Ulysses Duke Jenkins' *Ancient African Religion and the African-American Church* (1978) is about Yoruba religion. The book is inscribed "To Era Bell on her Birthday. Many happy, happy! With love, Louise 1979." Martin Ebon's *Maharishi, the Guru: An International Symposium* (1968) was source material for one of Thompson's articles, "Meditation Can Solve Race Problem," *Ebony* (May, 1968), pages 77-88. A photograph of Thompson and the Maharishi appear in *Ebony* (April, 1968), page 26. The Daughters of St. Paul's book *Visible Community of Love* (1969) has been annotated by Thompson. Marked are the sections on "Church, non-believers" and "Non-Christians." Also, there is Ted Patrick and Tom Dulack's *Let Our Children Go!* (1977), factual stories about Patrick's rescuing young people from religious sects.

The Vivian G. Harsh Research Collection's name for Thompson's personal library is the "Era Bell Thompson Collection in International Black Affairs." The name bespeaks a significant amount of travel and writing about international affairs. Altogether Era Bell Thompson did stories in Africa, India, Australia, South America, various islands in the South Pacific, and Israel. Examples of the latter include "Australia: its white policy and the Negro" (July 1956 and September 1956); "The smallest richest nation in the world" (May 1968), an article about the island country of Nauru in the South Pacific; and "The plight of black babies in South Vietnam" (December 1972).[12] One scholar mentions how influential these travelogues were to his choice of a college major in anthropology.[13]

Books in Thompson's library include atlases, travel guides, and books describing various aspects of the countries visited. Along with the *Rand McNally Collegiate World Atlas* (1961) and *Rand McNally Readers World atlas* (1965) are several Pan American Airways publications. Thompson has annotated the sections on Ghana, Guinea, Ivory Coast, Kenya, and Senegal in Pan American Airways' *New Horizons: The Guide to World Travel* (1954). Also annotated are *New Horizons U.S.A.: The Guide to Travel in the United States* (1967) and *Pan Am's World Guide: The Encyclopedia of Travel* (1974). The latter has markings for Barbados, Bermuda, Fiji Islands, New Zealand, Congo, Dahomey, and Kenya. Lastly, Marjorie Adoff Cohen's *Whole World Handbook: A Student Guide to Work, Study and Travel Abroad* (1976) has chapters on Western Europe, the U.S.S.R.

and Eastern Europe, the Middle East and North Africa, Africa south of the Sahara, South Asia (India, Nepal, Sri Lanka, Bangladesh, and Pakistan), East Asia, Southeast Asia, Australia and New Zealand, Latin America and the Caribbean, and Canada.

Several books about foreign countries are gifts from friends and associates. Among these are Richard Wright's *Black Power: A Record of Reactions in a Land of Pathos* (1954), inscribed by Adeline Pynchon "For Era Bell Thompson with love from her friend." The book is Wright's report on the revolution of Africa's Gold Coast. It has been annotated by Thompson. Waipuldanya and Douglas Lockwood's *I, the Aboriginal* (1965) is based on Lockwood's interviews with Phillip Roberts (Waipuldanya or Wadjiri-Wadjiri). It is has an inscription from Lockwood to Thompson. She has annotated the book and refers to it in her feature article "Part II. Australia: Its White Policy and the Negro," *Ebony* (September, 1966), page 102.

Halla Linker's *Three Tickets to Timbuktu* (1966) describes her travels in Peru and Bolivia, Nepal, Cambodia, South Africa, Ethiopia and Timbuktu. Richard B. Ford's *Tradition and Change in Four Societies: An Inquiry Approach* (1968) covers race relations, economic development, and totalitarism in Brazil, South Africa, India, and China. It includes a reprint of Era Bell Thompson's article "Does Amalgamation Work in Brazil?", *Ebony*, (July, 1965), pages 27-41. She has annotated a short section on black/white relations in rural and urban Australia in Craig McGregor's *Profile of Australia* (1967), pages 291-305. Anthony Howarth's *Kenyatta: A Photographic Biography* (1967) is inscribed by Abraham Boswel "For Era Bell Thompson to remind her of Kenya and of the enjoyment we shared in her own brave safari in Africa."

Books on international affairs include diplomat Pearl S. Buck's *My Several Worlds: A Personal Record* (1954), a gift from Adeline Pynchon inscribed "This book is a 'must' for your library – a great book by a great person." Born of missionary parents and brought up in China the author devotes the major part of this autobiography to a social and political description of China. Ronald Segal's book *The Race War* (1967) is annotated by Thompson. It discusses European and American exploitation of less developed countries, and political entrenchment along racial lines in relation to Russia and China. G. Mennen Williams' *Africa for the Africans* (1969) gives an account of his five-year service as Assistant Secretary of State for African Affairs. Thompson has underlined the sections on "Hope of a continent" and "Southern Rhodesia."

Thompson frequently attended book parties and author presentations convened by publishers. In a letter regarding a dinner held by the Society of Midland Authors, she writes "Last Monday night Dr. Joshua Loth Liebman, author of PEACE OF MIND, was a guest speaker at a dinner meeting of the Society of Midland Authors."[14] More routinely, she attended the book talks and receptions sponsored by the George K. Hall Library, a branch library in Chicago's black community.

The Hall Branch Library was both a base for Thompson's personal research and an outlet for meeting Chicago's literary and artistic community. Her ties to the Hall Branch Library spanned nearly 50 years. The inscription in her second book, *Africa: Land of My Fathers* (1954), reads "For the Hall Branch Library, where much of 'Land' was born and where 'American Daughter' took shape. I am most grateful to Miss Harsh and her staff for their kindness during my hours of strain and stress! Era Bell Thompson." Her volunteer service at the Library brought her into contact with many prominent authors, several of whom worked with the Federal Writers' Project of the Works Project Administration.

As a focal point for Chicago Renaissance writers and artists, the Hall Branch Library was a site for meetings, book talks and discussions, and a home for these intellectuals to engage in their research. The Library's "Special Negro Collection" was transferred to the Carter G. Woodson Regional Library in 1975 and renamed the "Vivian G. Harsh Research Collection of Afro-American History and Literature" in honor of the Hall Branch's long-term director. Among the writers and artists associated with the Hall Branch were Richard Wright, Arna Bontemps, Katherine Dunham, Margaret Walker, and Gwendolyn Brooks.[15]

Representative books by Chicago Renaissance writers in Thompson's library include Arna Bontemps' *We Have Tomorrow* (1945). The book is inscribed by the author to Thompson. It is a history of black role models that children and young adults can emulate. Bontemps and Jack Conroy's *They seek a city* (1945) is about rural-urban migration from the South. Conroy has inscribed the copy to Thompson. Sylvestre C. Watkins' *Anthology of American Negro Literature* (1944) is autographed by the author. Thompson has annotated the section of "Biographical notes." The Illinois Work Projects Administration's anthology *Cavalcade of the American Ne-*

gro (1940), edited by Arna Bontemps, is a history of black contributions to all phases of American life from 1865 to 1940.

Other books by Chicago Renaissance writers are Richard Wright's autobiographical novel *Black Boy: A Record of Childhood and Youth* (1945) as well as Thompson's classic autobiography *American Daughter* (1946). The autobiography covers her rise from a poverty stricken childhood, growing up in North Dakota, to becoming a senior interviewer with the United States Employment Service. Incidentally, Thompson's was featured among the authors and artists celebrated at the Jackson College Literary Festival (1952).[16] Margaret Walker's second book of poetry *Prophets for a New Day* (1970) is a collection of her civil rights poems written in response to the violence of the 1960s, including the bombing of the Sixteenth Street Baptist Church in Birmingham. Thompson has annotated this volume. Curiously, Walker's first book of poetry, *For My People* (1942), is not in the collection. There is no evidence it was ever owned by Thompson, but some literary critics consider it the most important collection of poetry by a Chicago Renaissance writer before Gwendolyn Brooks's *A Street in Bronzeville* (1945).[17]

There are quite a few gifts in the Thompson library. Of the 362 books in her collection, 37 are gifts or presentation copies from authors and friends. Documenting their long friendship, Gwendolyn Brooks has given Thompson numerous books. The following books are all inscribed by Brooks. *A Street in Bronzeville* (1945) describes a poetic walk through the Chicago black community reflecting the reality of oppression in the lives of urban blacks. The Pulitzer Prize for Poetry winner *Annie Allen* (1949) deals with three periods in a woman's life. *Maud Martha: A Novel* (1953) tells the story of a black girl growing to womanhood on Chicago's south side. *Bronzeville Boys and Girls* (1956) is a collection of poems inspired by Brooks' Chicago neighborhood.

Gwendolyn Brooks' *The Bean Eaters* (*1960*) includes 35 poems reflecting on the themes of prejudice, love, and hate with which African Americans are faced. *Selected Poems* (1963) contains poems from three earlier books: "A Street in Bronzeville," "Annie Allen," and "The Bean Eaters," as well as some new selections. *In the Mecca: Poems* (1968) contains a long narrative poem about a mother searching for her lost child in a Chicago apartment building and nine shorter poems based on contemporary figures and events. *Riot* (1969) is a poem in three parts that examines the social upheavals of the late 1960s. *Report from Part One* (1972) is an autobiography relating the events of Brooks' life to her ongoing struggle to freely express the ideas and emotions of an African American poet. And, lastly, Brooks' *The Tiger Who Wore White Gloves, or, You Are What You Are* (for children)(1974) is a collection of short stories in rhyme intended for juvenile audiences.

The Hall Branch Library regularly sponsored large community educational gatherings. Thompson's volunteer service at the Library specifically concerned selecting books and lecturers for the Book Review and Lecture Forum. Twice a month neighborhood residents gathered to hear book reviews or lectures followed by a discussion. Some of the Forum speakers were Zora Neale Hurston, Langston Hughes, Horace Cayton, and St. Clair Drake.[18]

Books by these speakers found in the Thompson library include Zora Neale Hurston's *Dust Tracks on a Road: An Autobiography* (1942), a book is about her rise from childhood poverty in the rural South to prominence as a leading intellectual of the Harlem Renaissance; Langston Hughes' *The Ways of White Folks* (1947), a series of short stories about social life, slavery, and racial passing. Hughes' *Simple Speaks His Mind* (1950) is a series of casual conversations to discuss issues of the day, mainly about race and racism. His *Something in Common and Other Stories* (1963) is a collection of 36 short stories. All three of the Langston Hughes' books are inscribed by the author to Thompson. St. Clair Drake and Horace R. Cayton's *Black Metropolis: A Study of Negro Life in a Northern City* (1962) is a historical and sociological account of Chicago's South Side covering rural-urban migration, community structure, and black-white race relations. The Thompson library also includes Cayton's autobiography *Long Old Road* (1965) which covers his friendship with prominent personages in politics and the arts such as Richard Wright and Sinclair Lewis.

In an effort to bring noted journalist Carl T. Rowan in as a Forum speaker, Ms. Thompson praises the Hall Library saying "we do have more pull and prestige than most organizations. We devote one or two nights a season to Negro authors and their books, a program which always rouses much community interest." In a follow-up letter to Rowan, she adds "Fletcher Martin is reviewing your book at the Library Forum November 5th. Would be wonderful if you could drop in. Think it would be possible?" [19]

Two of Rowan's books belong to the Thompson library. *South of Freedom* (1952) describes Rowan's 6,000 mile journey through the South to report on the reality of everyday life for blacks. The book is inscribed by Rowan to Thompson and announced in "Book of the Week," *Jet* (September 25, 1952), page 46. A second book by Rowan is *Just Between Us Blacks* (1974) which attacks white racism and criticizes blacks who fail to use the liberties and opportunities already gained. The book has an inscription to Thompson from Gwen Ifill who, in 1974, would have been an intern at the *Boston Herald-American*. This book was announced in "Books," *Jet* (December 26, 1974), page 55.

Tom Dent

Of the 1,477 books found in the Tom Dent library, 1,341 are included in this study. For the most part, only books by and about blacks and those which explore non-Western value systems have been selected.

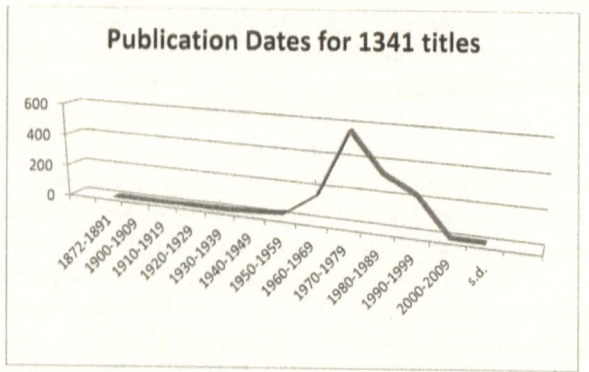

Figure 3: Publication Dates of Dent Collection Titles

Tom Dent's personal library includes several older publications. The collection includes 33 books published between 1872 and 1952. Some of the books have bookplates or inscriptions indicating prior ownership by Dent's parents. Dr. Albert W. Dent was the President of Dillard University in New Orleans. Mrs. Ernestine Jessie Covington Dent was a renowned concert pianist.[20] The books that are signed or book plated by the Dents are the *New Orleans City Guide* (1938), written and compiled by the Federal Writers' Project of the Works Progress Administration for the city of New Orleans. The book is signed "AW Dent." Worth Tuttle Hedden's novel *The Other Room* (1947) has the ownership stamp of Mrs. A.W. Dent. Langston Hughes' *New Negro Poets, U.S.A.* (1964) has Jessie Covington Dent's book plate. Tom Dent is one of 37 poets included the work.

Books given to both Mr. and Mrs. Dent include Brailsford R. Brazeal's *The Brotherhood of Sleeping Car Porters: Its Origin and Development* (1946) inscribed by "Bra" to Albert and Jessie Dent; and Faith Berry's *Langston Hughes, Before and Beyond Harlem* (1983), an examination of the poet's life and development of his writing. The book was a gift from Wallace and Henrietta Wells to Dr. and Mrs. Albert W. Dent. Other books were inscribed by their authors to Albert Dent singly. These include Langston Hughes' *One-Way Ticket* (1953), a collection of poetry; John D. Weaver's *The Brownsville Raid* (1973), about race relations and the dishonorable discharge of 167 black soldiers in the 25th Infantry Regiment; black college president Benjamin E. Mays' autobiography *Born to rebel* (1971); and *Louisiana's Black Heritage* (1979), a collection of conference papers presented at the Louisiana State Museum symposium held in New Orleans, April 15-16, 1977.

In addition to the three pre-1952 books already mentioned (Federal Writer's Project, 1938; Brazeal, 1946; and Hedden, 1947), there are 30 other books which were probably acquired by Tom Dent himself. Because some are stamped with the Congo Square writer's group imprint and/or were annotated by Dent, it is reasonable to suspect that he acquired them from second-hand and antiquarian bookstores. Among his 19th and early 20th century imprints are William Still's *The Underground Rail Road* (1872) which deals with antislavery movements; John B. Alden's *Alden's Handy Atlas of the World* (1889) with maps and statistics of all countries existing at the time; and Octavia V. Rogers Albert's *The House of Bondage* (1891), the result of a 13-year project interviewing former slaves. Dent has made annotations in this book. Booker T. Washington, N. B. Wood and Fannie Barrier Williams' *A New Negro for a New Century* (1900) is a collection of essays about the Spanish-American War, education, slavery, and the women's club movement; while Thomas Dixon's novel *The Clansman* (1905) is a story about the Ku Klux Klan during the Reconstruction era.

Pre-1953 literary works are Lafcadio Hearn and Albert Mordell's *An American Miscellany* (1924), vol. 2, an anthology of stories about creole language and literature, Voodoo, and Caribbean peoples; Margaret Walker's *For my people* (1942), a collection of poetry and lyrical ballads reflecting a strong folk tradition; M. W. Waters' drama *The Light-Ukukanya: a Drama of the History of the Bantus, 1600-1924* (1925) about blacks in South Africa; and Federico García Lorca's *From Lorca's Theatre: Five Plays of Federico Garcia Lorca* (1941); Edwin Honig's *García Lorca* (1944) is a biography about the playwright; Richard Wright's *Native son* (1940), a novel set in Chicago in the 1930s about a young black man caught in a downward spiral after he kills a young white woman in a brief moment of panic; and his *Uncle Tom's Children* (1943), a collection of short stories about race relations. The latter has the Congo Square writers' group ownership inscription. The Louisiana Writers' Project's *Gumbo Ya-Ya: A Collection of Louisiana Folk Tales* (1945) is a federal Works Progress Administration project.

Another book with the "Congo Square" inscription is Ralph Ellison's novel *Invisible Man* (1952), which is about a black man's fervent search for his identity. Lloyd L. Brown's *Iron City* (1951) is a prison novel about a black youth falsely convicted and sentenced to death for the murder of a white businessman; Alan Paton's *Cry, the Beloved Country* (1948), a South African novel about a black country parson whose son is condemned to hang for the murder of a white man. Dent has annotated this copy. Philippe Thoby-Marcelin and Pierre Marcelin's novel *The Beast of the Haitian Hills* (1946) tells the story of an urban storekeeper who moves to the countryside to make peace with his late wife, but comes to understand the reality of Voodoo.

Figure 3 depicts Dent's increased collecting activity from the mid-1950s through the mid-1960s. The uptick in acquisitions corresponds with his association with the Umbra writing workshop in New York and editorship of its literary magazine. This activity continues when he becomes Associate Director of the Free Southern Theater in New Orleans, establishes the BlackArtSouth writer's workshop and becomes editor of *Nkombo*, its literary magazine. Collection activity reaches its peak in the mid-1970s, corresponding with his founding the Congo Square writing group, his and Kalamu ya Salaam's transitioning of the *Nkombo* magazine into another New Orleans based magazine, the *Black Collegian*, and his co-founding and editing the first issue a new literary journal named *Cal-*

laloo (1976). His associates in the latter endeavor were Charles H. Rowell and Jerry W. Ward, Jr.

Issues concerning the the Free Southern Theater's sustainability formed the backdrop of an incident typifying Dent's fervor for collecting black books. While he advocated local performances coupled with book-oriented workshops, others preferred to continue grand tours throughout the South believing the emphasis on books and workshops misguided. Denise Nicholas, an actress who later starred in popular television series *Room 222* and *In the Heat of the Night*, believed the performances were the most effective way of educating a largely illiterate audience. "I know," she says, "that its essential non-literary form of communication (in the sense of people not having to know how to read to dig), its immediate contact, its liveliness, will beat books for centuries to come.... I have put my blinders back on—I only see theater...not books, but work, discipline." In the end the Theater's Board aligned with Dent, accepting his proposal to redirect the Theater's programming. He communicates this and the prospect of establishing a working library to Joe Goncalves, founder of the *Journal of Black Poetry* (1966). Dent writes "This summer we will not have a touring company, we will have a community workshop program in New Orleans: drama, writing, band, art, black history, current events. We will also have an Afro-American library of books and journals." [21]

Some eight years later, working with different writers group, Dent's resolve to develop a black heritage working library is equally fervent. He says to Charles Rowell, with whom he is preparing to solicit manuscripts for *Callaloo*, their new literary journal, "I want to use this spring to begin to look for monies.... We are looking for bread for the New Orleans journal, I'm also always looking for something for Congo Square to use for travel, like the Washington trip, and for the library, which we need badly." Months later this ambition is expressed to another colleague, "I want money for Congo Square to build an up-to-date library, but there just doesn't seem to be any except for jive projects." [22]

Apparently Dent's personal library initially was housed in the Free Southern Theater offices. He suggests, on more than one occasion, that materials from his collection were disappearing. He tells a colleague "listen, I thought I had the issue of *Rhythms* with the Skunder [Boghossian] display but I find I have two copies of the first issue. The issue you want is the second issue.... If I run across that second issue I'll send it to you, but it looks like someone picked it up." Another colleague writes to say "Somehow over the years I managed to run away with one of your books." [23]

The BlackArtsSouth and Congo Square writing groups each required source material for study, discussion and and performance. Dent helped to develop the collections of both organizations.[24] Eventually he would merge the two book collections into his own. Throughout this time his personal library remained open to friends and colleagues. Mildred Swift thanks him for showing her useful books by Blassingame and Christian in connection to her research project on Black women in Oklahoma. Robert Hemenway also expresses gratitude, writing "You were especially kind to trust me with your place—and your books—while you left for Atlanta." [25]

A number of books in the Dent library were acquired in order to write book reviews. For the most part, the review books were supplied by editorial departments and publishers seeking to publicize their products. Dent reviewed books for *Freedomways* from 1970 until 1985. The journal ceased publication in 1985. He reviewed books for the *Black American Literature Forum* from 1979 to 1992. He also wrote book reviews for the *American Book Review*, the *Black Scholar*, *Southern Exposure*, and *South and West: An International Literary Quarterly*.[26]

Often Dent would contact book review editors asking if they were interested in having a given book evaluated. Many times those editors with whom he had established good working relations would solicit reviews from him. As a freelance writer Dent was paid for his work. Payment for the reviews supplemented his salary from the Free Southern Theater. Because of the many essays and book reviews he had written for *Freedomways* magazine, he was invited to join their staff as a Contributing Editor. He was expected to write several essays and/or book reviews a year. Presumably he would continue to receive payment from the magazine. Among the many publishers supplying Dent with free books were the Bobbs-Merrill Co., William Morrow and Co., Longman Pub., University of California Press, and University of Tennessee Press.

A major influence on Dent's intellectual development was Barbadian poet, prose writer, and historian Dr. Edward Kamau Brathwaite. Brathwaite was a founding member of the Caribbean Arts Movement (1966) and editor of its journal, *Savacou*. The two poets shared correspondence and books. While an adjunct professor at the University of New Orleans,

Dent received funding from the Committee on Lecturers and Artists to sponsor Brathwaite's campus visit.[27]

An intriguing group of letters that Brathwaite sent Dent concerned the former's home and damaged personal library. Michael E. Paty, a project manager with the United Nations Development Program assigned to the University of the West Indies, writes an unflattering letter about Brathwaite's home and library and challenges Brathwaite to take responsibility for his own neglect. He writes: "Your personal house ... is in poor condition. Damage to the badly designed house was aggravated by the hurricane. In the house is kept your superb collection of books, which I have had the pleasure of seeing for myself." Handwritten commentary by Brathwaite run throughout the letter, questioning Paty's veracity almost line by line. Included with the Paty letter is a copy of the one-page letter of rejoinder by Brathwaite to the University's Vice Chancellor. It is unclear whether the library was saved. Years later Dent had the opportunity to participate on a panel at a the Kamau Brathwaite and the Caribbean Word: North-South Counterpoint conference held at Hostos Community College, City University of New York, October 24, 1992.[28]

Several poetry books authored by Brathwaite are inscribed to Dent. These are *Mother poem* (1977); an 8-page poem *Word Making Man: Poem for Nicolás Guillén in Xaymaca* (1979); *Soweto* (1979), another 8-page poem; *Middle Passages* (1992) includes poems "How Europe underdeveloped Africa" and "Soweto"; and *Barabajan Poems, 1492-1992* (1994). Poetry books that were not inscribed are *Masks* (1968); *Shar* (1990), also called *Hurricane Poem*; *Third World Poems* (1983), a complimentary copy from Brathwaite's publisher; and *Trench Town Rock* (1994), a collection of visual poetry.

Other works in the Dent library Brathwaite's *Contradictory Omens: Cultural Diversity and Integration in the Caribbean* (1974), inscribed to Tom Dent; *DreamStories* (1994), a collection of short stories inscribed to Tom Dent; *Roots: Essay* (1986), a collection of literary criticism appearing between 1957 and 1979; and Brathwaite's 12-page work of criticism and interpretation entitled *Jerry Ward & the Fragmented Spaceship Dreamstory* (n. d.). Books about history and black folk culture include Brathwaite's *Nanny, Sam Sharpe, and the Struggle for People's Liberation* (1977); *The Folk Culture of the Slaves in Jamaica* (1981); and a biography *The Zea Mexican diary, 7 Sept 1926-7 Sept 1986* (1993), about his wife Doris Monica Brathwaite who died of cancer. The book is inscribed to Dent.

Dent's library includes Doris Monica's bibliography *EKB, His Published Prose & Poetry, 1948-1986: A Checklist* (1986) which Dent has annotated; J. F. Ade Ajayi and Sidney Wilfred Mintz' *Slavery, Colonialism, and Racism* (1974) which include Brathwaite's "The African presence in Caribbean literature"; and Gordon Rohlehr's *The Shape of that Hurt and Other Essays* (1992) which features several essays about Brathwaite. These are "Megalleons of light: Edward Brathwaite's Sun poem," "Brathwaite with a dash of brown: crit, the writer and the written life," and "The rehumanization of history: regeneration of spirit, apocalypse and revolution in Brathwaite's The arrivants and X/Self." Rohlehr inscribes the book to Dent and Dent has annotated it.

Dent's interest in African history and culture was honed by another important protege/mentor relationship. He maintained a close relationship with South African poet and political activist Keorapetse Kgositsile. In 1960s Kgositsile was recognized as one of the Black Arts Movement's central poets. Pulitzer Prize winner Gwendolyn Brooks pays homage to him in her poem "Young heroes: To Keorapetse Kgositsile (Willie)" in *Family Pictures* (1970). She also writes the introduction to his well-regarded poetry collection *My Name is Afrika* (1971). Both books are in the Dent library.

Kgositsile mentored Dent as the latter harbored an ambition to succeed as poet. When Dent was admitted to graduate school at Goddad College (Vermont), he asked Kgositsile to serve on his graduate committee. Dent was admitted to Goddard's low residency graduate program and was therefore able to continue work in New Orleans at the Free Southern Theater. In his capacity as editor of *Nkombo* magazine, Dent invited Kgositsile to New Orleans as a resource person. "We are asking," Dent writes, that you help us with completion of a special poetry issue, and with a program that we are putting together for Black History Week in conjunction with the Free Southern Theater." Eager that his poetry capture Africa's significance as a point of reference for evaluations about black life and culture, Dent asked his mentor to recommend a list of ten essential books on African history and culture. We were unable to find a record of which books Kgositsile recommended. In Fall, 1974, Dent earned his master's degree in poetry.[29]

Several books in the Dent Library are inscribed to Dent from "Willie," as Kgositsile is also known. These are *My Name is Afrika* (1971); *The Word Is Here: Poetry from Modern Africa* (1973); *When the Clouds*

Clear (1990); *The Present Is a Dangerous Place to Live* (1993); and *To the Bitter End* (1995). Also in the collection, but not inscribed, are *Places and bloodstains: Notes for Ipelang* (1975) and *Approaches to Poetry Writing* (1994). The latter is annotated by Dent. Anthologies with essays by Kgositsile include Patricia L. Brown, Don L. Lee and Francis Ward's *To Gwen with Love: An Anthology Dedicated to Gwendolyn Brooks* (1971), inscribed by Gwendolyn Brooks to Dent; Stephen Evangelist Henderson's *Understanding the New Black Poetry: Black Speech and Black Music as Poetic References* (1973), inscribed by the author to Tom Dent; and Gwendolyn Brooks' *A Capsule Course in Black Poetry Writing* (1975).

Supplementing publishers' catalogs and review media such as the *American Book Review*, Dent relied on social networks established from his days with the Umbra, BlackArtsSouth, and Congo Square writing groups. Dent and his associates maintained contact with one another, writing regularly from the late 1960s through the 1990s. For instance, in the 1970s Ishmael Reed recommends new books by LeRoi Jones and Ernest Gaines, *Tales* (1967) and *The Autobiography of Miss Jane Pittman* (1971) respectively. Onita Marie Hicks tells Dent about Ishmael Reed's the *Yardbird Reader* special issue on "Black Pre-History" guest-edited by John A. Williams and about Wilfred Cartey's new book of Trinidadian poetry *Suns and Shadows* (1978).

In the 1980s Jerry Ward shares information about James Baldwin's *The Evidence of Things Not Seen* (1985), a small essay on the Atlanta child murders, and *The Price of the Ticket: Collected Nonfiction 1948-1985* (1985), a collection of Baldwin's nonfiction writings. He also alerts Dent to William J. Harris' new book *The Poetry and Poetics of Amiri Baraka: The Jazz Aesthetic* (1985). Calvin Hernton tells Dent about a new book by Clarence Majors titled *My Amputations* (1986), which is the first novel written Majors in the ten years since his *Reflex and Bone Structure* (1976).

In the 1990s Marita Rivero recommends Henry Louis Gates' autobiography *Colored People: A Memoir* (1994); Sara Lawrence-Lightfoot's *I've Known Rivers: Lives of Loss and Liberation* (1994), a biography of six middle-class African Americans; and James McBride's autobiography *The Color of Water: A Black Man's Tribute to His White Mother* (1996); and Charles Payne informs Dent that John Dittmer's book *Local People: The Struggle for Civil Rights in Mississippi* (1994) will be out in the spring.[30]

Notes

1. Thomas Covington Dent Papers. Amistad Research Center, Tulane University. New Orleans, Louisiana. Miscellaneous. Personal Financial Records, Bank Statements & Checks. Series VIII. Box 225; Letter to My brother Willie, 6/2/80. O.Correspondence, 1980. Box 25: Folder 4; and Letter from Roy Lewis, 2-7-81. Correspondence, 1981 Feb.; Box 9: Folder 2. Dent's Southern Black Cultural Alliance, together with the Southern Collective of African-American Writers and the Committee on Black South Literature and Art, received a $10,000 National Endowment for the Humanities award (Grant number: GP-*0475-81) for the Conference on Black Literature and Arts, November 20-22, 1980, at Emory University.

2. Ben Burns Papers, Vivian G. Harsh Research Collection of Afro-American History and Literature,Chicago Public Library, http://www.chipublib.org/cplbooksmovies/cplarchive/ archivalcoll/ burns.php.; and Burns, Ben. *Nitty Gritty: A White Editor in Black Journalism*. Jackson, MS: University Press of Mississippi, 1996, p. 11.

3. Janega, James. "Ben Burns, 86, White Editor Who Made Mark In Black Journalism." *Chicago Tribune*, (February 2, 2000), p. 2C8; and Golden, Harry. "How to Get Rich." *Chicago Daily Defender* (April 18, 1970), p. 8.

4. Burns, Ben. *Nitty Gritty: A White Editor in Black Journalism*. Jackson, MS: University Press of Mississippi, 1996, pp. xii, and 14.

5. Ibid., p. 30.

6. Ibid., p. 35.

7. Joyce, Donald Franklin. "Black Bibliophiles and Collectors: Preservers of Black History" in *College & Research Libraries*, May 1991, p. 302. Donald Franklin Joyce. *Black Book Publishers in the United States. A Historical Dictionary of the Presses, 1817-1990*. New York: Greenwood Press, 1991.

8. DeFreece-Wilson, Eileen, "Era Bell Thompson: Chicago Renaissance Writer," p. 182.

9. Thompson, Era Bell, *American Daughter*, p. 197.

10. Thompson's non-Johnson Publishing Company eviews found in the Era Bell Thompson Papers. Box 7. Folder: Book Reviews. Specific titles of the transcribed radio programs are: Thompson, Era Bell. "The Teen Age Book

Parade." Review of *My Antonia*. By Willa Cather. Continuity from Broadcast Music, Inc., 1951. 5p. Number TBP-26. Transcript of a radio broadcast (time: 14:30). Thompson, Era Bell. "The Book Parade." Review of *The Sojourner* by Majorie Kinnan Rawlings. Continuity from Broadcast Music, Inc., 1955. 4p. Number BP-206. Transcript of a radio (time: 14:30); and Thompson, Era Bell. "The Book Parade." Review of *The Muses are heard by Truman Capote*. Continuity from Broadcast Music, Inc., 1957. 4p. Number BP-320. Transcript of a radio broadcast (time: 14:30).

11. Era Bell Thompson Papers. Letter from Langston Hughes to Era Bell Thompson, August 19, 1957. Box 7. Folder: Book Reviews.

12. DeFreece-Wilson, Eileen, "Era Bell Thompson: Chicago Renaissance Writer," p. 163.

13. Boyd, Alex. "A Select Six Anthropologists." *The Network Journal*, May 10, 2011 Url: http://www.tnj.com/black-history-makers/select-six-black-anthropologists (last accessed: 2/19/13).

14. Era Bell Thompson Papers. Correspondence. Box 12. Folder 53. Letter from Mrs. Richard Bokum, June 29. Box 12. Folder 53. Bokum writes "I'm so glad you were here for the Harper party"; and Letter from Era Bell Thompson to Mr. Porterfield, May 17, 1948. Box 10 Pasquetti-Stille. Folder: Society of Midland Authors.

15. DeFreece-Wilson, Eileen, "Era Bell Thompson: Chicago Renaissance Writer," p. 24.

16. Ibid., p. vi.; p. 17; p. 26.

17. Hine, Darlene Clark, William C. Hine, and Stanley Harrold. *The African American Odyssey*. Upper Saddle River, NJ: Prentice Hall, 2011, p. 522.

18. Burt, Laura. "Vivian Harsh, Adult Education, and the Library's Role as Community Center." *Libraries & the Cultural Record*, 44, no. 2 (2009): 240.

19. Era Bell Thompson Papers. Letter from Era Bell Thompson to Carl Rowan, July 8, 1952; Era Bell Thompson Papers. Correspondence. Box 10. Folder: Rowan, Carl. Correspondence. Box 10. Rowan, Carl. Letter from Era Bell Thompson to Carl Rowan, September 24, 1952.

20. Lundy, Anne and and Ernestine Jessie Covington Dent. "Pioneer Concert Pianist." *The Black Perspective in Music* Vol. 12, No. 2 (Autumn, 1984), pp. 244-265].

21. Thomas Covington Dent Papers, Amistad Research Center, Tulane University. Letter from Denise Nicholas, June 16, 1967. Correspondence, 1967. Box 1: Folder 10; and Letter to Joe Goncalves, 18 May 30, 1968. O.Correspondence, 1955-56, 1966-67. Box 24: Folder 2.

22. Ibid. Letter to Charles Rowell, 1/22/76. O.Correspondence, 1976. Box 24: Folder 16; and Letter to Onita [Marie Hicks], 4/10/76. O.Correspondence, 1976. Box 24: Folder 16.

23. Ibid. Letter to Doris. June 8, 1971. O.Correspondence, 1971 Jan-June. Box 24: Folder 8; and Letter from Marion (M.K.M.). 4/27/83. Correspondence, 1983 April. Box 11: Folder 1.

24. A partial list of records (invoices, bookstores, and titles purchased) for the BlackArtsSouth library are in Nkombo Publications records, Amistad Research Center at Tulane University, New Orleans, Louisiana. Nkombo Publications. Correspondence-Bookstores, 1969. Box 1: Folder 14 through Folder 16. A partial list of Congo Square library books and borrowers from 1976 through 1978 is in the Thomas Covington Dent Papers, Amistad Research Center, Tulane University. Series 5: Project Files, 1966-1998. Box 188: Folder 8: Congo Square Writers Association: library loan lists, 1976-1978.

25. Thomas Covington Dent Papers, Amistad Research Center, Tulane University. Letter from Mildred Swift, 12-16-80. Correspondence, 1980 December. Box 8: Folder 16; and Letter from Robert Hemenway, May 27, 1981. Correspondence, 1981 May. Box 9: Folder 5.

26. Correspondence about book reviews for *Freedomways* in the Thomas Covington Dent Papers. See Letter to Esther Jackson, December 8, 1970. Series I: O.Correspondence, 1970 July-Dec. Box 24: Folder 27; Letter from Esther Jackson, July 18, 1978. Correspondence, 1978 July. Box 6: Folder 15; Letter from Esther Jackson, April 21, 1980. Correspondence, 1980 March. Box 8: Folder 8; Letter from Esther Jackson, February 25, 1981. Correspondence, 1981 February. Box 9: Folder 2; and Letter from Esther Jackson, January 11, 1985. Correspondence, 1985 January. Box 12: Folder 4.

Correspondence from the *Black American Literature Forum* include Letter from Joe Weixlmann, April 19, 1979. Correspondence, 1979 April. Box 7: Folder 8; Letter from Joe Weixlman, Oct. 21, 1982. Correspondence, 1982 Oct. Box 10: Folder 13; Letter from M. Alam, September 24, 1984. Correspondence, 1984 September. Box 11: Folder 18; Letter from Henry Louis Gates, Jr., November 7, 1986. Correspondence, 1986 Nov. Box 13:

Folder 7; and Letter from Keith Byerman, 24 August 1992. Correspondence, 1992 August Box 19: Folder 6.

Correspondence regarding the *American Book Review* include Letter from Suzanne Zavrian, 7/12/78. Correspondence, 1978 July. Box 6: Folder 15; and Letter from Bert Part, 5/31/89. Correspondence, 1989 May. Box 16: Folder 5. Several references to other review media for whom Dent wrote reviews are found at Letter from Janice Bevien for the Editors/*Black Scholar*, March 26, 1980. Correspondence, 1980 March. Box 8: Folder 7; Letter from Marc Miller, *Southern Exposure,* September 1, 1983. Correspondence, 1983 September. Box 11: Folder 6; and Letter from Pinkie Gordon Lane, *South and West: An International Literary Quarterly*, 1/4/79. Correspondence, 1979 Jan. Box 2: Folder 5.

27. Ibid. Letter from Kamau, 10 July 1978. Correspondence, 1978 July. Box 6: Folder 15]; and Letter from Anthony G. Tassin, April 30, 1979. Correspondence, 1979 April. Box 7: Folder 8.

28. Ibid. Letter to Professor E. Brathwaite from Michael E. Paty (3 pages), March 15, 1989. I. Correspondence. Box 16: Folder 3.

29. Ibid. Letter to Mr. Keorapetse Kgositsile, February 18, 1974. O. Correspondence, 1974. Box 24: Folder 14; Letter to Willie, 11/30/73. O. Correspondence, 1973-Dec. Box 24: Folder 13; and Letter from Craig (Graduate College), October 14, 1974.

30. Notifications from friends about new books are found in the Thomas Covington Dent Papers, Amistad Research Center, Tulane University. Letter from Ishmael Reed, December 9, 1967. Correspondence, 1967 July-Dec. Box 1: Folder 11; Letter from Ishmael Reed, October 3, 1970. Correspondence, 1970 July-Dec. Box 2: Folder 6; Letter from Peter Nazareth, May 13, 1978. Correspondence, 1978 May. Box 6: Folder 13; Letter from Onita Marie Hicks, December 3, 1978. Correspondence, 1978 Dec. Box 7: Folder 4; Letter from Jerry Ward, October 13, 1985. Correspondence, 1985 Oct. Box 12: Folder 13; Letter from Jerry Ward, January 28, 1986. Correspondence, Jan. 1986. Box 13: Folder 1; Letter from Calvin Hernton, Nov. 23, 1986. Correspondence, 1986. May. Box 13: Folder 5; Letter from Gilbert Fletcher, 4-19-92. Correspondence, 1992 April. Box 19: Folder 2; Letter from Marita Rivero, June 24, 1994. Correspondence, 1994 June. Box 21: Folder 3, Letter from Marita Rivero, Friday 9, 1994. Correspondence, 1994 September. Box 21: Folder 6; Letter from Marita Rivero, 5/6/98. Correspondence, 1998 May. Box 23: Folder 4; and Letter from Charles Payne, October 11, 1993. Correspondence, 1993 October. Box 20: Folder 7.

Chapter Four

Text Network Analysis

Consider a scenario in which the networks of book collectors consist of subject, geographical, and various other terms and phrases descriptive of their individual books. Think of the terms and phrases as nodes in a network of bibliographic descriptors. The nodes themselves are a step removed from the content they describe which, in turn, affect a collector's thoughts about social and cultural realities. Within their networks nodes have relative degrees of importance. Some have comparatively high degree centrality because they frequently link to other nodes in the network. The importance of some is measured by their closeness or average distance from other nodes. While others still are important because they hold pivotal positions between many pairs of nodes.

Method

In this chapter the major components of the Burns, Thompson and Dent libraries are identified as network nodes. Both the important nodes and their relationships to other nodes are analyzed. The data for this study is derived from the bibliographic records of books in the three personal libraries. Except for subject descriptors, all other bibliographic detail was removed. The descriptors themselves are based on Library of Congress Subject Headings (LCSH), a controlled vocabulary. Several modifications to the original subject headings have been made. Chief among these is that complex phrases are reduced to simpler components. For example, the LCSH phrase *Negro Leagues—History—Juvenile Literature* is parsed into smaller terms and phrases: *Negro Leagues*, *History*, and *Juvenile Literature*.

Certain words are treated as "stop words" and were omitted because they occur in the LCSH phrases too frequently. These include "African American," "Literature," and "United States." Another modification is that several concepts are subsumed under broader concepts. For example, "Interracial sex" is used in place of "Interracial dating," "Interracial marriage," "Miscegenation," "Mixed-race people," "Racially mixed persons," and "Passing (identity)." Also, rather than list the names of specific cities, states, countries, etc., broader geographic terms are used such as "Midwestern states," "Southern states," "Africa," "Caribbean area," and "South America." Although works of fiction generally are not assigned LCSH descriptors, in some cases themes gleaned from summaries of works were added to their subject fields.

After eliminating stop words, the next-most frequently occurring terms were manually detected by perusing the list of descriptors. All subject fields not containing one or another of these descriptors were eliminated. The remaining descriptors were manually keyed into Microsoft Excel spreadsheets. These in turn were imported into a software tool called *Gephi*, an open-source graph visualization and exploration platform for all kinds of networks.[1] *Gephi* also provides metrics for analyzing the modularity (community structure) and relationships between nodes such as distance and betweenness.

Results

Based on the list of modified LCHS terms, the 12 most frequently occurring terms in the Burns library are "Africa," "Caribbean area," "Interracial sex," "Slavery," "History," "Race relations," "Southern states," "Autobiography," "Juvenile literature," "Jazz music," "Fiction," and "Biography." These, together with adjacent terms, were input into a Microsoft Excel worksheet. The results, formatted as Excel CVS worksheets, were then imported into the Gephi software tool. Modularity measures the division of a network into modules (i.e., groups, clusters, or communities). Nodes within a given cluster have dense connections, but are sparsely linked to the nodes of other clusters. The modularity algorithm included in Gephi's statistics and metrics framework reveals seven clusters in the Burns network. The size of these particular clusters are 52, 33, 82, 42, 62, 63, and 51 nodes each.

The nine most prevalent terms are in descriptive of Era Bell Thompson's library are "Race relations," "Biography," "Africa," "Midwestern states," "Poetry," "Autobiography," "Civil rights," "History," and "Southern states." The Gephi modularity algorithm establishes that there are seven clusters in this network. The sizes of the clusters are 32, 92, 30, 52, 20, 33, and 48 nodes, respectively.

The fifteen most predominant descriptors of the Dent library are "Civil rights," "Race relations," "Autobiography," "Biography," "Africa," "Caribbean area," "Southern states," "Slavery," "Women," "Anthologies," "Authors," "Poetry," "History," "Fiction," and "Jazz music." Gephi calculates that the Dent network is comprised of eight clusters. The sizes of these clusters are 126, 52, 100, 51, 83, 74, 226, and 100 nodes, respectively.

Node Cluster Groupings

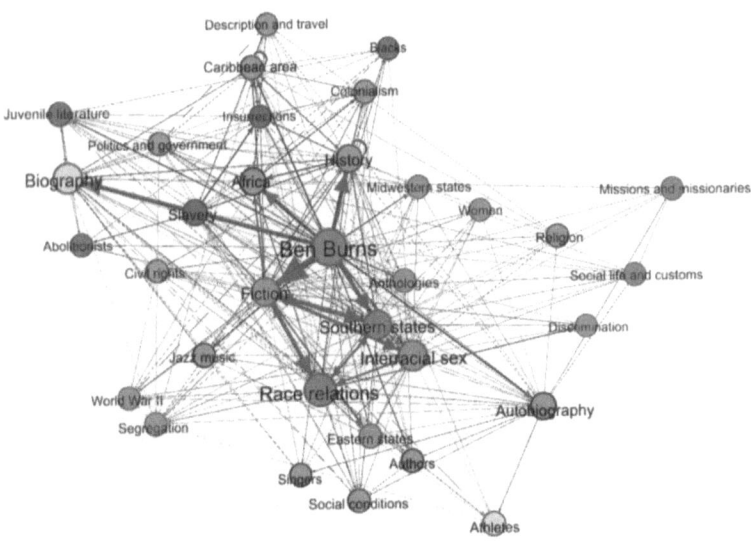

Figure 4: Burns Network Graph

Figure 4 above represents the Burns network. The nodes are represented by circles and the connections between them denoted by lines and arrows called edges or links. Nodes with fewer than 23 edges were filtered out. The graph displays five of the six clusters in the Burns network. Group one includes "Race relations" and "Southern states." Group two includes "Biography" and "Athletes." Group three has "Fiction," "Anthologies," "Interracial sex," "Eastern states," "Midwestern states," and "Segregation." Group four has "Juvenile literature," "Slavery," and "Insurrections." Group five contains "Jazz music," "Africa," "Social conditions," "Autobiography," "History," "Colonialism," and "Caribbean area."

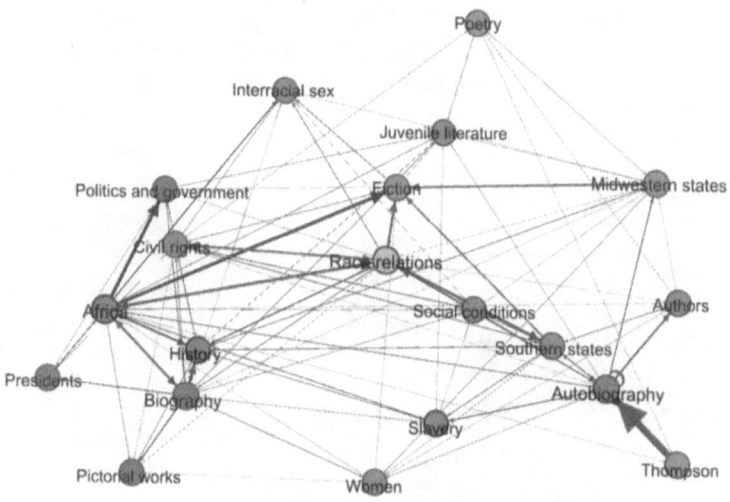

Figure 5: Thompson Network Graph

The Thompson network is represented by Figure 5. Nodes with fewer than eight edges have been filtered out. Five of the seven clusters identified by Gephi are displayed. Group one includes "Poetry," the sole node in the cluster with a degree ranking of eight or higher. Group two contains "Biography," "Politics and government," "Presidents," and "Pictorial works." Group three has "Southern states," "Social conditions," "Autobiography," "Authors," and "Juvenile literature." Group four has "Civil rights," "Interracial sex," "Fiction," "Women," and "Midwestern states." Group five has "Africa," "History," and "Slavery."

THOMAS WEISSINGER

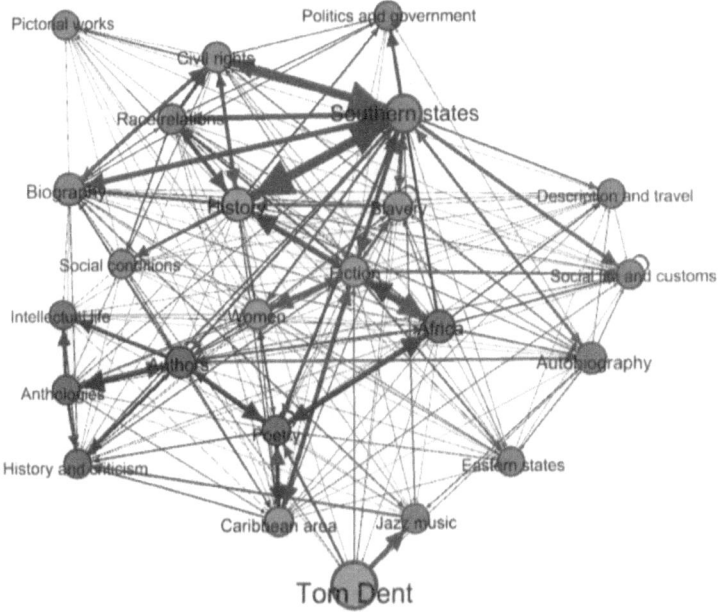

Figure 6: Dent Network Graph

The Dent network is illustrated by Figure 6. Nodes with fewer than 27 links were filtered out. Five of the seven clusters comprising this network are represented. Group one contains "History," the only node in the cluster with a degree rank of 27 or higher. Group two includes "Southern states," "Pictorial works," "Social conditions," "Description and travel," "Social life and customs," and "Eastern states." Group three includes "Race relations," "Biography," "Politics and government," "Autobiography," and "Jazz music." Group four has "Africa," "Poetry," "Authors," "Intellectual life," "History and criticism," and "Anthologies." Group five has "Civil rights," "Women," "Slavery," "Fiction," and "Caribbean area."

Degree Centrality

Degree centrality can be defined as the number of connections a node has to other nodes. The more connections a node has, the greater its degree of centrality in a network. The 19 most connected nodes in each the Burns and Thompson networks, and 20 most connected in the Dent

Ben Burns network	Era Bell Thompson network	Tom Dent network
Africa (81 links)	Africa (102 links)	Africa (167 links)
Anthologies (24)	Authors (21)	Anthologies (59)
Athletes (25)	Autobiography (80)	Authors (133)
Autobiography (93)	Biography (70)	Autobiography (163)
Biography (141)	Civil rights (42)	Biography (189)
Caribbean area (55)	Fiction (31)	Caribbean area (93)
Colonialism (24)	History (35)	Civil rights (122)
Eastern states (30)	Interracial sex (14)	Description & travel (31)
Fiction (138)	Juvenile literature (15)	Eastern states (44)
History (108)	Midwestern states (45)	Fiction (157)
Insurrections (27)	Pictorial works (13)	History (220)
Interracial sex (91)	Poetry (13)	History & criticism (54)
Jazz music (30)	Politics & govt (15)	Jazz music (55)
Juvenile literature (49)	Presidents (12)	Poetry (95)
Midwestern states (24)	Race relations (86 links)	Politics & govt (34)
Race relations (139 links)	Slavery (16)	Race relations (122)
Segregation (27)	Social conditions (17)	Slavery (80)
Slavery (71)	Southern states (45)	Social conditions (46)
Social conditions (28)	Women (15)	Social life & customs (43)

Southern states (118)		Southern states (309)
		Women (89)

Figure 7: Degee Centrality

network, are displayed in Figure 7.

For the Burns network "Biography" has the highest degree centrality. In the Thompson network "Africa" ranks highest. "Southern states" ranks highest in the Dent network.

Closeness Centrality

Closeness centrality is a measure of the average distance between pairs of nodes in a network. High closeness centrality means that the average path distance between nodes is relatively far. A low closeness centrality means the average distance between pairs of nodes is relatively short. In social networks closeness centrality is sometimes described in terms of degrees of separation or the portion of all others an actor can reach (influence, control, etc.) in one, two, three steps, etc.[2] Nodes with relatively short average path distances represent adjacency between information content and ideas of value to a book collector, while those with longer average path distances are more marginal.

The average distance between pairs of nodes in the Burns network is 3.27. Figure 8 lists nodes in the network with average path lengths of 2.70 (or less). The average distance between pairs of nodes in the Thompson network is 3.54. Nodes with average paths of 2.99 (or less) are listed in Figure 8. The average path between pairs of nodes in the Dent network is 3.19. Nodes with an average path of 2.65 or less are listed below.

Ben Burns network (N= 2.70 or less)	**Era Bell Thompson Network** (N= 2.99 or less)	**Tom Dent network** (N= 2.65 or less)
Abolitionists (2.61 rank)	Africa (1.70 rank)	Africa (1.89 rank)
Africa (1.88)	Athletes (2.71)	Anthologies (2.32)
Anthologies (2.54)	Authors (2.28)	Authors (1.95)

Armed forces (2.62)	Autobiography (1.82)	Autobiography (1.93)
Authors (2.40)	Biography (1.93)	Bibliographies (1.00)
Autobiography (1.99)	Civil rights (2.06)	Biography (1.86)
Biography (1.73)	Description & travel (2.20)	Caribbean area (2.21)
Blacks (2.51)	Economic conditions (2.78)	Civil rights (2.20)
Caribbean area (2.04)	Fiction (2.21)	Dictionaries & encyclopedias (2.25)
Civil rights (2.62)	History (2.10)	Discrimination (2.65)
Colonialism (2.51)	Housing (2.78)	Education (2.63)
Discrimination (2.60)	Juvenile literature (2.99)	Fiction (1.87)
Eastern states (2.53)	Midwestern states (2.05)	Folklore (2.64)
Economic conditions (2.66)	Missions & missionaries (2.65)	History & criticism (2.49)
Education (2.66)	Nationalism (2.44)	History (1.80)
Fiction (1.82)	Pictorial works (1.33)	Insurrections (2.61)
Foreign relations (2.62)	Poetry (2.58)	Jazz music (2.36)
History (1.80)	Presidents (2.45)	Poetry (2.02)
History & criticism (2.54)	Race relations (1.79)	Politics & govt (2.58)
Insurrections (2.54)	Rural-urban migration (2.86)	Presidents (2.65)
Interracial sex (1.86)	Segregation (2.78)	Race relations (2.19)

Jazz music (2.16)	Social classes (2.20)	Reconstruction (2.59)
Juvenile literature (2.00)	Social conditions (2.69)	Revolutions (2.64)
Lynching (2.62)	South America (2.00)	Riots (2.61)
Midwestern states (2.61).	Southern states (2.25)	Segregation (2.62)
Missions & missionaries (2.54)	Africa (1.70)	Sexual abuse (2.47)
Passing (identity) (2.56)		Short stories (2.62)
Race relations (1.83)		Slavery (1.98)
Reconstruction (2.57)		Social conditions (2.61)
Religion (2.58)		Social life & customs (2.65)
Rural-urban migration (2.67)		Soldiers (2.64)
Segregation (2.48)		South America (1.00)
Short stories (2.43)		Southern states (1.78)
Slavery (1.88)		Women (2.21)
Social conditions (2.50)		
Social life & customs (2.38)		
Southern states (1.82)		
World War II (2.67)		

Figure 8: Closeness Centrality

Betweenness Centrality

Betweenness centrality is based on the number of shortest paths between any two nodes that pass through a particular node. It measures how often a node appears on the shortest paths between pairs of nodes. A high betweenness centrality may indicate that a node bridges together disparate clusters in a network. The removal of such a node may mean that the nodes or clusters it had formerly connected would now stand in isolation. The total number of shortest paths in the Ben Burns network is 118044. There are 29658 shortest paths in the Thompson network and 551952 in the Dent network. Figure 9 lists nodes with the highest betweenness centrality rankings for each of the three networks.

Ben Burns network (31 highest betweenness centrality rankings)	**Era Bell Thompson network** (36 highest betweenness centrality rankings)	**Tom Dent network** (41 highest betweenness centrality rankings)
Abolitionists (2015 rank)	Abolitionists (699 rank)	Africa (62591 rank)
Africa (12094)	Africa (8949)	Anthologies (8904)
Anthologies (3761)	Anti-apartheid movements (229)	Athletes (3926)
Athletes (4877)	Athletes (689)	Authors (49423)
Authors (2922)	Authors (2713)	Autobiography (48974)
Autobiography (10929)	Autobiography (6115)	Biography (55983)
Biography (19249)	Biography (4045)	Blues music (2266)
Caribbean area (4670)	Blacks (534)	Caribbean area (23409)
Civil rights (1978)	Caribbean area (229)	Children (2064)

Clergy (1254)	Church (476)	Civil rights (27320)
Colonialism (2865)	Civil rights (2947)	Civilization & culture (6519)
Dictionaries & encyclopedias (1181)	Clergy (649)	Clergy (2530)
Eastern states (4116)	Diplomats (694)	Criticism & interpretation (5626)
Economic conditions (1203)	Discrimination (283)	Description & travel (4856)
Fiction (14985)	Fiction (2081)	Discrimination (2364)
History (12281)	Foreign relations (904)	Eastern states (9055)
Insurrections (1670)	Freedmen (460)	Fiction (41271)
Interracial sex (19246)	Gospel music (479)	Folklore (4180)
Jazz music (4040)	History (3769)	History (84550)
Juvenile literature (4204)	Interracial sex (573)	History & criticism (12591)
Midwestern states (1845)	Juvenile literature (1834)	Insurrections (4611)
Missions & missionaries (1813)	Lynching (596)	Jazz music (14935)
Politics & govt (2029)	Midwestern states (5660)	Labor unions (2456)
Race relations (25620)	Missions & missionaries (492)	Midwestern states (3570)
Religion (2361)	Native Americans (691)	Native Americans (3873)
Segregation (1978)	Physicians (1033)	Pictorial works (7101)

Slavery (8521)	Poetry (866)	Poetry (21057)
Social conditions (3221)	Politics & govt (646)	Politics & govt (8391)
Social life & customs (1793)	Presidents (951)	Race relations (26257)
Southern states (16857)	Race relations (8110)	Religion (2096)
World War II (1652)	Singers (460)	Slavery (24144)
	Slavery (2277)	Social conditions (11392)
	Social conditions (981)	Social life & customs (6550)
	Southern states (4624)	Soldiers (2555)
	United Nations (904)	Southern states (141684)
	Women (906)	Southwestern states (3570)
		Underground railroad (3348)
		Vietnam War (6187)
		Voter registration (3327)
		Western states (2172)
		Women (26821)

Figure 9: Betweennness Centrality

Discussion

The nodes which Gephi groups into clusters appear to have a "family resemblance" because they tend to be about the same kinds of thing, i.e., literature, race relations, social conditions, and so on. As such, the connections between nodes in a cluster are apparently conceptually related. However, in some instances the family resemblance is not so obvious. For example, in the Burns network the nodes "Interracial sex," "Segregation," and "Jazz music," appear somewhat out of place given the clusters to which they are assigned. Recall that "Interracial sex" and "Segregation" are in Group three of the Burns network, along with "Fiction," "Anthologies," and regional descriptor s for Eastern and Midwestern sections of the United States. "Jazz music" is in Group five with "Africa," "Social conditions," "Autobiography," "History," "Colonialism," and "Caribbean area."

On the surface the placement of "Jazz music" in Group five is counter-intuitive. However, there is a reasonable explanation; namely that the linkages between subject matter owe to shared content or associations. Because "immersion in the Negro world" encompassed reverence for black music and musicians, Burns and his wife frequented the jazz clubs of Chicago.[3] While on sabbatical in Paris, the couple occupied themselves with "evenings of casual club crawling" around Parisan nightspots. Jazz bands were models of integrated society, often interracial in composition. In Paris luminaries such as Sidney Bechet and Bricktop had become popular postwar fixtures. Bechet was a black clarinetist and saxophonist, Ada "Bricktop" a black singer/dancer and night club owner. White clarinetist Mezz Mezzrow, whom Burns claims "passed as a Negro in the jazz world," often visited the Burns' Parisan apartment.[4]

It also seems counter-intuitive that "Interracial sex" and "Segregation" are in Group three. An explanation is that such unlikely pairings are bridged by nodes denoting genres. For example, Groups three and five include the genre nodes "Hstory," "Autobiography," "Fiction," and "Anthology." Note the high betweenness centrality metrics for the first three nodes, ranking 12281, 10929, and 14985, respectively. While the betweenness rankings of the last genre node is low in comparison at 3761, "Anthology" ranks higher in betweenness centrality than most subject nodes. Rather than say that "Jazz music," "Interracial sex," and "Segregation" have poor family resemblances with other nodes in their clusters, the idea to take away from this is that subject nodes with high betweenness centrality bridge node pairs in a cluster together. They have some elements in common with other nodes, but otherwise may be quite different.

Another example of a genre node that bridges disparate subject matter can be seen in Group four of the Burns network, regarding the relation between "Juvenile literature," "Slavery," and "Insurrections." The upshot of this is that "Juvenile literature" does a serviceable job conveying information about slavery and abolitionist movements, even though other genre may also effectively treat the subject matter. Books written for young adults may have plotlines about historical material just as "Fiction," "History," and "Autobiography" may capture the essence of social and economic conditions such as 20th century patterns of rural-urban migration of blacks from southern to northern states ("Midwestern states" and "Eastern states").

On the whole, three categories of node were found in the Burns, Thompson, and Dent networks. There are nodes about subjects (particular persons, topics, or events), nodes about genre (autobiography, fiction, anthologies, and juvenile literature, poetry, folklore, pictorial works, etc.), and geographical nodes. What clues do the node configurations and categories provide with respect to building a functional African American personal library? Taken as a whole, the centricity metrics are somewhat prescriptive. To start with, genre nodes which rank highest in closeness centrality are "Anthologies," "Autobiography," "Biography," "Fiction," "History," "History and criticism," "Juvenile literature," and "Poetry." "History and criticism" indicate books of interpretation and criticism from an arts and literature standpoint. With the exception of "History and criticism," all of these genre nodes rank high betweennness centrality.

In all three personal libraries, genre, perhaps more than any other category, make these libraries functional. Not only do the genres package and disseminate ideas in different ways, they suggest different ways of absorbing information. For instance, historical, autobiographical, or fictionalized narratives may rely on the same data, but use different methods, writng conventions, and standards of authenticity. While historical works make informed judgments based on primary sources, autobiographical and fictionalized works have more freedom to embellish. In autobiography an event may be mis-recollected, in historical fiction it is subject to artistic license.

Several geographic nodes rank high in closeness centrality. As mentioned earlier, nodes named for cities, states, countries, etc., are subsumed under broader geographic denotations such as "Eastern states," "Midwestern states," "Southern states," "Southwestern states," "Western states." "Africa," "Caribbean area," "South America," and "Central America." "Description and travel" is also applicable as a geographic term since it is about the cultural and physical geography of a place. Less obvious as geographic nodes are "Blacks" and "African Americans." Recall that the descriptors used in this study are derived from Library of Congress subject headings (LCSH). In LCSH "Blacks" and "African Americans" both refer to black people, but separates them based on their locations. The former denotes the black populations of the Caribbean, South America, Africa, Europe, and elsewhere. "African Americans" designates the black population of the United States. "African Americans" would be a major node in all three networks (Burns, Thompson, and Dent), but is excluded as a stop word. "Blacks," on the other hand, has a strong closeness centrality ranking in all three networks. Its average path length in Burns, Thompson, and Dent is 3.02, 2.05, and 2.74, respectively.

Figure 8 is a list of the highest ranking subject nodes in the three networks. All of nodes have strong closeness centrality metrics. The short path distances between these and other network nodes indicate significant and substantial relationships. Some subjects are important to all three bibliophiles. These are "Race relations," "Authors," "Social conditions," "Segregation," and "Civil rights." A second group of subjects are important to only two out of three book collectors. These are "Jazz music," "Slavery," "Social life and customs," "Missions and missionaries," "Insurrections," "Discrimination," "Economic conditions," "Education," and "Presidents." The remaining subjects in Figure 8 had importance to a singular bibliophile.

The subjects in Figure 8 can be reasonably arranged into eight categories. The categories are Art and Culture, Political Affairs, Human Rights, International Affairs, Race Relations, Social Life and Customs, and Social Conditions. The categories themselves have an enduring quality. On the other hand, the importance of any given topic which they categorize may be temporal, depending on the make-or-break matters of the day.

The category Art and culture includes "Jazz music," "Authors," "Athletes," and "Women." Social life and customs includes "Religion," "Rural-urban migration," and "Social life & customs." Included under

Social conditions are "Social classes," "Social conditions," "Segregation," "Discrimination," "Economic conditions," "Education," "Housing," and "Sexual abuse (domestic violence)." The category International affairs contains "Colonialism," "Missions & missionaries," "Foreign relations," and "Presidents." The category Human rights includes "Civil rights," "Nationalism," "Revolutions," and "Insurrections." Political Affairs includes "Presidents" and "Politics & government." Social movements includes "Civil rights," "Abolitionists," "Antislavery movements," "Riots (urban)," and "the Reconstruction era." Race relations categorizes "Interracial sex" (and related nodes such as miscegenation, biracial identity, interracial dating, etc.), "Passing (identity)," "Lynching," "Soldiers," "Armed forces," and "World War II."

Some subject nodes belong to more than one category. For instance, "presidents" covers presidents of African countries such as William V. S. Tubman, Idi Amin, and Kwame Nkrumah as well as American presidents Franklin Roosevelt, Harry S. Truman, and John F. Kennedy. Both the Burns and Thompson libraries include Irving Wallace's novel about a fictitious black president who is impeached by the U. S. Senate. "Insurrections" denote slave rebellions in the United States and elsewhere; as well as rebellions against British Loyalists and supporters of colonial rule.

While subject matter is of utmost importance, a mere collection of best books does not constitute a working personal library. Generalizing from the categories and network structures of the Burns, Thompson, and Dent libraries, it is clear that a good African American personal library should at least include important subject, genre, and geographical nodes. Putting the categories and central nodes together, a functional personal library might take the following form. Apart from serving as a heuristic device, the following list has the advantage of citing books which were selected and actually used in African American personal libraries.

Genre Categories
Anthologies

1. Brown, Patricia, Don L. Lee and Francis Ward. *To Gwen with Love: An Anthology Dedicated to Gwendolyn Brooks*. Chicago: Johnson Pub. Co., 1971. 149p. Announced in "Ebony Book Shelf," *Ebony*, April 1971, p. 26. Initial idea of the tribute came from the Kuumba Workshop, a group of Chicago artists who were personally acquainted with Brooks. Includes poems and prose contributions from all over the country. (Thompson collection; also a copy inscribed by Brooks in the Dent collection)

2. Davis, Arthur P. and Michael W. Peplow. *New Negro Renaissance: An Anthology*. New York: Holt, Rinehart & Winston, 1975. 538p. A thematically arranged collection of short selections and excerpts from the fiction, nonfiction, poetry, and drama of famous and lesser-known black American writers active between 1910 and 1940. (Burns collection)

3. Ajayi, J. F. Ade, Sidney Wilfred Mintz, et al. *Slavery, Colonialism, and Racism*. Boston: American Academy of Arts and Sciences, 1974. 205p. Contains 11 essays by twelve contributors dealing with Africa and the African diaspora in the United States, the Caribbean and Latin America. Partial content include: The Black experience of colonialism and imperialism by Philip D. Curtin; The Caribbean region by Sidney W. Mintz; The African presence in Caribbean literature by Edward Kamau Brathwaite; Black Africa: the historians' perspective by J. F. Ade Ajayi and E. J. Alagoa; Themes in African literature today by Per Wastberg; Black history unbound by Benjamin Quarles. (Dent collection)

Autobiography

1. Taylor, Susie King. *A Black Woman's Civil War Memoirs: Reminiscences of My Life in Camp with the 33rd U.S. Colored Troops, Late 1st South Carolina Volunteers*. New York: M. Wiener Pub.; dist. by the Talman Co., 1988. 154p. Originally published in 1902 as *Reminis-*

cences of My Life in Camp with the 33d United States Colored Troops, Late 1st S.C. Volunteers. Annotated. Content: A brief sketch of my ancestors; My childhood; On St. Simon's Island, 1862; Camp Saxton--proclamation and barbecue, 1863; Military expeditions, and life in camp; On Morris and other islands; Cast away; A flag of truce; Capture of Charleston; Mustered out; After the war; The Women's Relief Corps; Thoughts on present conditions; A visit to Louisiana. (Dent collection)

2. Redding, J. Saunders. *On being Negro in America.* Indianapolis: Bobbs-Merrill, 1951. 156p. Review copy from publisher. Annotations in the form of vertical line markings in margins. Reviewed in "Book of the Week," Jet, November 1, 1951, p. 56. Writes about his personal life covering various themes from days as a part-time Communist, Garveyism, and defense of interracial marriage. (Burns collection)

3. Brooks, Gwendolyn. *Report from Part One.* Detroit: Broadside Press, 1972. 215p. Annotations in the form of horizontal line markings. Inscribed by the author to Thompson. Exerpt included in *Ebony*, March 1973, pp. 115-120. Relates the events of her life to her ongoing struggle to freely express the ideas and emotions of an African American poet. (Thompson collection)

Biography

1. Bontemps, Arna. *100 Years of Negro Freedom.* New York: Dodd, Mead, 1961. 276p. Included among "Top Ebony Bookshop Sellers," *Jet*, December 13, 1962, p. 26. Focuses on scientists, educators, and politicians who have struggled to bring freedom and equality to blacks in the century following the Emancipation Proclamation. (Thompson collection)

2. Spritzer, Lorraine Nelson and Jean B. Bergmark. *Grace Towns Hamilton and the Politics of Southern Change.* Athens, GA: University of Georgia Press, 1997. 253p. Annotated. Content: Genesis; Growing up Negro in the progressive era; A rude awakening in Ohio; The depression years: to Memphis and back; The emerging

leader; The Atlanta Urban League: a housing success; At the AUL: equalizing funds for Negro schools and the rebirth of Negro voting; A hospital for the excluded and the "hidden agenda"; A leave and a resignation; Hamilton and the civil rights movement; The lady from Fulton; The years of racial solidarity; Waning solidarity, growing power; A landslide defeat; The last years. (Dent collection)

3. Rogers, J. A. *World's Great Men of Color*. New York: Macmillan, 1972. 2 vols. Content: Vol. 1. Asia and Africa, and historical figures before Christ, including: Akhenaton, Aesop, Hannibal, Cleopatra, Zenobia, Aakia the Great, the Mahdi, and Samuel Adjai Crowther. Vol. 2. Europe, South and Central America, the West Indies, and the United States, including: St. Benedict the Moor, Alessandro de Medici, Aleksander Pushkin, Joachim Murat, Alexandre Dumas, Dom Pedro II, Robert Browning, and Marcus Garvey. (Burns collection)

Dictionaries and Encyclopedias

1. Bailey, Leaonead Pack. *Broadside Authors and Artists: An Illustrated Biographical Directory*. Detroit: Broadside Press, 1974. 125p. Includes bio-bibliographies of 192 persons. Out of a total of 183 entries for Americans, 169 (94%) are not listed in *Who's Who in America 1972-1973*. (Dent collection)

2. Murray, Florence. *The Negro Handbook (1944)*. New York: Current Books, 1944. 283p. Various "lists and digests make this book a compendium of facts on outstanding events in Negro life. …The compilation of such detailed work is no easy task and Miss Murray is to be congratulated on having brought it to the point of clear, orderly and expeditious arrangement. " –Dorothy Porter, *Journal of Negro Education* 12 (Spring 1943), p. 221. (Burns collection)

3. Salk, Erwin A. *A Layman's Guide to Negro History*. Chicago: Quadrangle Books, 1966. 170p. Announced in "Books Noted," *Negro Digest*, September 1966, p. 93. Inscribed "Personal property of E. B. T." Includes a suggested basic library of black history, information about organizations, inventions, important dates, early

black petitions and protests, black congressmen, population census figures, and so on. (Thompson collection; also a copy in the Burns collection)

Fiction

1. Bontemps, Arna Wendell. *Black Thunder*. Boston: Beacon Press, 1968. 224p. The slave Gabriel can no longer abide bondage and seizes upon Old Testament promises of God's vengeance against evil and rallies his fellow slaves for freedom. They plot to kill the white people in Richmond in hopes of fostering a general black uprising. In the end a betrayed Gabriel dies calmly on the gallows. (Dent collection)

2. Motley, Willard. *We Fished All Night*. New York: Appleton-Century-Crofts, 1951. 560p. Burns ownership inscription. Review copy from publisher. Highlighted in "Books," *Jet*, January 31, 1952, p. 57 as "rambling story of three confused, groping youths of the foundering 40s." Motley, a black novelist from Chicago, writes about three white veterans in post-war Chicago. Liberal Jim Norris, Jewish and mentally ill Aaron Levin, and Don Lockwood, a Polish American war hero. Motley's emphasis on universality and the near absence of African Americans as major characters in his work placed him in the company of several gifted African American authors who flirted with *"raceless"* or *"assimilationist fiction"* in the 1940s and 1950s. (Burns collection)

3. Petry, Ann. *Tituba of Salem Village*. New York: Crowell, 1964. 254p. Announced in "Ebony Book Shelf," *Ebony*, November 1964, p. 26. Tells how Tituba, a slave, was sold in Barbados to a preacher bound for Boston and became one of three women convicted at the beginning of the Salem witch trials. (Thompson collection)

Folklore

1. Felton, Harold W. *John Henry and His Hammer*. New York: Knopf, 1950. 82p. Burns ownership inscription. Describes the life

of the legendary African American hero who was born and who died with a hammer in his hand. (Burns collection)

2. Hughes, Langston and Arna Bontemps. *The Book of Negro Folklore*. New York: Dodd, Mead, 1958. 624p. One of ten bestsellers for sale through the "Ebony Bookshop" buy-by-mail order plan, *Jet*, Janaury 29, 1959, p. 54. Content: Animal tales; Animal rhymes; Memories of slavery; Sometimes in the mind; God, man and the devil; Do you call that a preacher?; Ghost stories; Black magic and chance; On the levee; Amen corner; Spirituals; Gospel songs; Pastime rhymes; Ballads; Blues; Work songs; Street cries; Playsongs and games; The jazz folk; Harlem jive; The "problem"; Songs in the folk manner; Poetry in the folk manner; Prose in the folk manner. (Thompson collection)

3. Louisiana Writers' Project. *Gumbo Ya-Ya: A Collection of Louisiana Folk Tales*. Compiled by Lyle Saxon, Edward Dreyer and Robert Tallant. New York: Bonanza Books, 1945. 581p. Material gathered by workers of the Works Progress Administration, Louisiana Writers' Project, and sponsored by the Louisiana State Library Commission. Content: Kings; Baby dolls; Zulus; and Queens; Street criers; The Irish Channel; Axeman's jazz; Saint Joseph's day; Saint Rosalia's day; Nickel gig, nickel saddle; The Creoles; The Cajuns; The temple of innocent blood; The plantations; The slaves; Buried Treasure; Ghosts; Crazah and the glory road; Cemeteries; Riverfront lore; Pailet lane; Mother Shannon; The sockserjaise gang; Songs; Chimney sweeper's holiday; A good man is hard to find; Who killa da chief?; Superstitions; Colloquialisms; Customs. (Dent collection)

History

1. Bernal, Martin. *Black Athena: The Afroasiatic Roots of Classical Civilization*. New Brunswick, NJ: Rutgers University Press, 1987. Dent Collection has vol. 1 of the 3 volume set. Annotated. Argues that classical Greek civilization had deep roots in Afro-asiatic cultures. Content: v. 1. The fabrication of ancient Greece, 1785-1985. (Dent collection)

2. Bohannan, Paul and Philip Curtin. *Africa and Africans.* Garden City, NY: Published for the American Museum of Natural History by Natural History Press, 1971. 391p. Rev. ed. Covers the great empires, slavery, colonial government, art, family life, religion, economy and policy. (Thompson collection)

3. Williams, John A. *Africa: Her History, Lands and People Told with Pictures.* New York: Cooper Square Publishers, 1962. 128p. John A. Williams was a correspondent for *Ebony* and *Jet* magazines. book contains several hundred pictures and 25,000 words. Partial content include: A highlight chronology of events and dates; The Egyptian dynasties; The Greeks, Romans, Persians and Chinese in ancient Africa; The great ancient African empires; The African slave trade in the new world; European conquest; Colonization and development in Africa; Ancient and recent maps. (Burns collection)

Juvenile Literature

1. Du Bois, Shirley Graham. *Your most Humble Servant: The Story of Benjamin Banneker.* New York: Messner, 1949. 235p. Biography of Benjamin Banneker, eighteenth-century Negro, whose almanac, inventions, contributions to the planning of Washington, D.C., and letter to Thomas Jefferson on the right of Negroes made him a distinguished citizen in American history. (Burns collection)

2. Bontemps, Arna Wendell. *Story of the Negro.* New York: Knopf, 1948. 239p. Inscribed by the author to Era Bell Thompson. Annotations in the form of horizontal line markings. Reviewed by Thompson in June 13, 1948 *Chicago Sun-Times.* [Also, Eileen DeFreece-Wilson cites a letter from Bontemps thanking Thompson for a favorable review, "Era Bell Thompson: Chicago Renaissance Writer," Ph.D. thesis, p. 108.] History of blacks from early civilizations in Africa through the practice of slavery in many areas, especially the United States, to early twentieth century achievements of African Americans. (Thompson collection)

3. Katz, William Loren. *Black Indians: A Hidden Heritage.* New York: Atheneum, 1986. 198p. Annotated. Traces the history of

relations between blacks and American Indians, and the existence of black Indians, from the earliest foreign landings through pioneer days. (Dent collection)

Pictorial Works

1. Editors of Ebony. *Ebony Pictorial History of Black America*. Chicago: Johnson Pub. Co., 1971. 4 vols. Written by the editors of Ebony and coordinated by historian and senior editor Lerone Bennett Jr. Content: v. 1. African past to the Civil War; v. 2. Reconstruction to Supreme Court decision 1954; v. 3. Civil rights movement to Black revolution; v. 4. The 1973 year book. (Thompson collection)

2. Hughes, Langston and Milton Meltzer. *A Pictorial History of the Negro in America*. New rev. ed. New York: Crown, 1963. 337p. Review copy from publisher. Annotated by means of a handwritten enclosure with instructions about the layout of a review article with photographs, presumably for *Sepia* magazine. Covers African American life from pre-revolutionary times to the civil rights movement. (Burns collection; also the Dent collection has a copy of the 3rd edition)

3. Smith, Michael P. *Spirit World: Pattern in the Expressive Folk Culture of Afro-American New Orleans*. Gretna, LA: Pelican Pub. Co., 1992. 120p. Originally published in 1984 by the New Orleans Urban Folklife Society. Inscribed by the author to Tom Dent. An exhibition and catalog sponsored by the Louisiana State Museum and the Amistad Research Center under a major grant by the Louisiana Committee for the Humanities. (Dent collection)

Poetry

1. Hughes, Langston. *Montage of a Dream Deferred*. New York: Holt, 1951. 75p. Review copy from publisher. Comprised 91 individually titled poems intended to be read as a single long poem. "[T]his poem on contemporary Harlem, like be-bop, is marked by

conflicting changes, sudden nuances, sharp and impudent interjections, broken rhythms, and passages sometimes in the manner of a jam session, sometimes the popular song, punctuated by the riffs, runs, breaks, and disc-tortions of the music of a community in transition." –L. Hughes. Subject: Poetry; Jazz music (Be-bop). (Thompson collection)

2. Pool, Rosey E. *Beyond the Blues: New Poems by American Negroes*. Lympne, Kent: Hand and Flower Press, 1962. 188p. Includes works of African American poets Leslie M. Collins, Paul Veasey, Gwendolyn Brooks, Countee Cullen, Langston Hughes, and Sterling Brown. (Burns collection)

3. Hughes, Langston. *New Negro poets, U.S.A.* Bloomington, IL: Indiana University Press, 1964. 127p. Book plate of Jessie Covington Dent. Reviewed by Dent (Thomas Covington Dent Papers. Series 2: Box 41. Folder 14). Compiles some 90 poems by a total of 37 poets. Poets include LeRoi Jones, Margaret Danner, Gloria Oden, Conrad Kent Rivers, Naomi Long Madgett, James A. Emanual, Mari Evans, Audrey Lorde, Dudley Randall, Tom Dent, David Henderson, and Calvin C. Hernton. (Dent collection)

Short Stories

1. Baraka, Imamu Amiri. Tales. New York: Grove Press, 1968. 132p. collection of short stories. The stories are "'fugitive narratives' that describe the harried flight of an intensely self-conscious Afro-American artist/intellectual from neo-slavery of blinding, neutralizing whiteness, where the area of struggle is basically within the mind," Robert Elliot Fox wrote in *Conscientious Sorcerers: The Black Postmodernist Fiction of LeRoi Jones/Baraka, Ishmael Reed Collection of Short Stories*. The stories are "'fugitive narratives' that describe the harried flight of an intensely self-conscious Afro-American artist/intellectual from neo-slavery of blinding, neutralizing whiteness, where the area of struggle is basically within the mind," Robert Elliot Fox wrote in *Conscientious Sorcerers: The Black Postmodernist Fiction of LeRoi Jones/Baraka, Ishmael Reed* (*Conscientious Sorcerers, and Samuel R. Delany.*, and Samuel R. DelanyGreenwood Press,

1987). (Dent collection)

2. Colter, Cyrus. *The Beach Umbrella*. Iowa City, IA: University of Iowa Press, 1970. 225p. Inscribed by the author to Thompson. Annotation in the form of a check mark in margin on page 207. Announced in "Ebony Book Shelf," *Ebony*, September 1970, p. 24. Chicago Settings for the stories range from ghetto existence to the *élite monde* of the Hyde Park-Kenwood black community. *The Beach Umbrella* was selected by novelists Vance Bourjaily and Kurt Vonnegut, Jr. to receive the first *Iowa School of Letters Award for Short Fiction*. Content: A man in the house; A chance meeting; The rescue; The lookout; Girl friend; Rapport; Mary's convert; Black for dinner; Moot; Overnight trip; An untold story; After the ball; A gift; The beach umbrella. (Thompson collection)

3. Hughes, Langston. *Something in Common, and Other Stories*. New York: Hill & Wang, 1963. 236p. Inscribed by the author to Burns. Thirty-seven short stories chosen by Hughes to present a cross section of his work as a short-story writer. (Burns collection)

Geographic Categories
Africa

1. Hopkinson, Tom. *In the Fiery Continent*. Garden City, NY: Doubleday, 1963. 367p. Annotations in the form of horizontal line markings. Announced in "Ebony Book Shelf," *Ebony*, July 1963, p. 24. A leading London journal tells of experiences in Africa when he was editing *Drum* magazine. To work for white South Africans with black South Africans, treating them as equals, says Hopkinson, was like balancing on knife-edge. (Thompson collection)

2. Legum, Colin. *Africa Handbook*. Rev. ed. Hammondsworth, England: Penguin Books, 1969. 681p. Reference book covering countries of Africa with essays, maps, political, information, and biographical information. (Burns collection)

3. Davidson, Basil. *The Search for Africa: History, Culture, Politics*. New York: Times Books, 1994. 373p. Annotated. Content: Thinking About Africa; Claims. The Search for Africa's Past. Africa

and the Invention of Racism. Rescuing Africa's History. Africanism and Its Meanings; Antipathies. Race and Resistance. The Roots of Antiapartheid. South Africa: A System of Legalized Servitude. African Saga. Pluralism in Colonial African Societies; Sympathies. African Peasants and Revolution. Voices from the Front. The Legacy of Amilcar Cabral; Debates. Nationalism and Its Ambiguities. Nationalism and Africa's Self-Transformation. The Politics of Restitution. Southern Africa: Progress Or Disaster?; Arguments. The Ancient World and Africa: Whose Roots? The Curse of Columbus. (Dent collection)

Caribbean Area

1. Lansing, Marion Florence. *Liberators and Heroes of the West Indian Islands.* Boston: L. C. Page, 1953. 294p. Reviewed in "Book of the Week," *Jet*, April 16, 1953, p. 50. Includes chapters on the most important Afro-Caribbean people such as Christophe, Dessalines, Petion, Marti, and Toussaint. (Burns collection)

2. Dunham, Katherine. *Island Possessed.* Garden City, NY: Doubleday, 1969. 280p. Katherine Dunham received a Rosewald Fellowship to study both dance and ritual in the Caribbean and Brazil in 1936. She found in Haiti endless variations of her two interests and revisited the country numerous times. (Thompson collection)

3. Dathorne, O. R. *Dark Ancestor: The Literature of the Black Man in the Caribbean.* Baton Rouge: Louisiana State University Press, 1981. 288p. Inscribed by the author to Andrew Young   Content: Africa as source; Oral literature and the reality of Africa; Africa affirmed in Afro-American literature; Responses to Africa; Contact, conflict, and reconciliation; Afro-New World movements: Harlem Renaissance, Negrista, and Negritude; The black puriverse; Towards synthesis: an opinion. (Dent collection)

Central America

1. Aveni, Anthony F. *Skywatchers of Ancient Mexico.* Austin, TX:

University of Texas Press, 1980. 355p. Presentation copy from Gilbert Fletcher. Thomas Covington Dent Papers, Amistad Research Center, Tulane University. Letter from Gilbert Fletcher, 7/23/81. Correspondence, 1981. July. Box 9: Folder 7. Gilbert writes "I found it, this was the last copy of Skywatchers and it wasn't even on the shelf. ...Why the interests in ancient astrology. What's in here that you are searching for." (Dent collection)

2. Muntslag, F. H. J. Tembe and Hein Eersel. *Surinaamse Houtsnijkunst. Suriname Wood-Carving. Symboliek van de Meest Voorkomende Motieven. Symbolism of the Most Frequent Motifs*. Amsterdam, The Netherlands: Herengracht 284, Prins Berhard Fonds, 1966. 64p. Gift of the staff of the Torarica Hotel in Suriname. (Thompson collection)

3. Wilson, Charles Morrow. *Empire in Green and Gold: The Story of the American Banana Trade*. New York: H. Holt, 1947. 303p. The public relations director of the United Fruit Company writes about the development of banana agriculture in Central America and the Caribbean from the early days of bartering by Cape Cod skippers to the organized monopoly of the United Fruit Company. (Burns collection)

Description and Travel

1. Matthiessen, Peter. *African Silences*. New York: Random House, 1991. 225p. Annotated. Author's account of his travels in Western Africa in 1978 and in Eastern Africa in 1986 tells of the vanishing worlds of Africa and what is replacing them. (Dent collection)

2. Robeson, Eslanda Goode. *African Journey*. New York: John Day Co., 1945. 154p. Inscribed by the author to Burns. Mrs. Robeson finds the familiar patriarchical attitudes in South African whites, the problems of segregation and discrimination, and an increased interest by blacks of international politics. Subject: Africa; Description and travel. (Burns collection)

3. Thompson, Era Bell. Africa: land of my fathers. Garden City, NY:

Doubleday, 1954. 281p. Inscribed "For the Hall Branch Library, where much of 'Land' was born and where 'American Daughter' took shape. I am most grateful to Miss Harsh and her staff for their kindness during my hours of strain and stress! Era Bell Thompson." The editor of *Ebony* magazine spent 3 months touring 18 countries on the African continent. (Thompson collection)

Eastern States

1. Anson, Robert Sam. *Best Intentions: The Education and Killing of Edmund Perry*. New York: Random House, 1987. 221p. Annotated. Journalist Anson explores how Edmund Perry, a 17 year old black honors student from Harlem, was killed soon after graduation by a young white plain clothes policeman in an alleged mugging attempt. (Dent collection)

2. Thomas, Will. *The Seeking*. New York: A. A. Wyn, 1953. 290p. Burns ownership inscription. Reviewed in "Book of the Week," *Jet*, June 11, 1953, p. 38. Thomas is a former journalist. He tells of moving his family to Vermont to live in an old farm house and how an all-white community accepted a black family into its social fabric. (Burns collection)

3. Brown, Claude. *Manchild in the Promised Land*. New York: New American Library, 1965. 429p. Review copy from publisher. Autobiographical novel of life as young black male coming of age amidst poverty and violence in Harlem during the 1940s and 1950s. (Thompson collection; also copy in the Dent collection)

Midwestern States

1. Cortesi, Lawrence. *Jean duSable: Father of Chicago*. Philadelphia: Chilton Book Co., 1972. 177p. Biography of the black Haitian who was the first non-Native American to settle and establish a trading community on the site of present day Chicago. (Burns collection)

2. Dawley, David. *A Nation of Lords: The Autobiography of the Vice Lords*. Garden City, NY: Anchor Press, 1973. 200p. About one of one of Chicago's largest street gangs and its transformation into a community organization dedicated to economic and social development. (Dent collection)

3. Thompson, Era Bell. *American Daughter*. Chicago: University of Chicago Press, 1946. Inscribed by Thompson to her brother Stewart. Ms. Thompson received a Fellowship in Midwestern Studies from the Newberry Library in 1945 to write her classic autobiography. Covers rise from a poverty stricken childhood, growing up in North Dakota, to becoming a senior interviewer with the United States employment service. (Thompson collection; copy also in the Burns collection)

South America

1. Freyre, Gilberto. *Brazil: An Interpretation*. New York: Knopf, 1945. 179p. Annotations in the form of vertical line markings in margins. Emphasizes heterogenous ethnic and cultural influences, including racial intermixture of European whites, Africans, and Native Americans, that distinguish Brazil from the other countries of South America. (Burns collection)

2. Pierson, Donald. *Negroes in Brazil, a Study of Race Contact at Bahia*. Chicago: University of Chicago Press, 1942. 392p. Annotations in the form of horizontal line markings. Winner of the John Anisfield Awards in Racial Relations in 1942 (announced in *Negro Digest*, vol. 1, p. 24). At the time written, this and Arthur Ramos' *The Negro in Brazil*, 1939, were practically the one literature on the subject in English. (Thompson collection)

3. Branch, Taylor and Eugene M. Propper. *Labyrinth*. New York: Viking Press, 1982. 623p. "How a stubborn U.S. prosecutor penetrated a shadowland of covert operations on three continents to find the assassins of Orlando Letelier"--Jacket subtitle. Letelier a Chilean lawyer, economist, politician and diplomat, was an outspoken critic of the Pinochet regime from exile. He was assas-

sinated in Washington, D.C. in 1976. The investigation uncoverd the existence of Operation Condor, which helped the governments of Chile, Argentina, Brazil, Uruguay, Paraguay and Bolivia capture one another's rebels and dissidents. (Dent collection)

Southern States

1. Redding, J. Saunders. *No Day of Triumph*. New York: Harper & Bros., 1942. 342p. Introduction by Richard Wright. Bookplate of Era Bell Thompson. Tells how, with funds provided by the Rockefeller Foundation and the University of North Carolina, Mr. Redding set out on an automobile trip through black America to see how people lived in the South. On December 3, 1943, Redding was awarded the Mayflower Cup by North Carolina Society of Mayflower Descendants for the best book written by a resident of the state. He was the first African American to win the award. (Thompson collection)

2. Naipaul, V. S. *A Turn in the South*. London: Viking, 1989. 307p. Content: Down home: A landscape of small ruins; Atlanta: Tunning in; Charleston: The religion of the past; Tallahassee: The truce with Irrationality; Tuskegee: The truce with irrationality; Jackson, Mississippi: The frontier, the heartland; Nashville: Sanctities; Chapel hill: Smoke. (Dent collection)

3. Woodward, C. Vann. *The Strange Career of Jim Crow*. Rev. and enl. ed. New York: Oxford University Press, 1957. 183p. Burns ownership inscription. Definitive study of racial segregation in the United States. Presents evidence that segregation in the South dated only to the 1890s.; that even under slavery, the two races had not been divided as they were under the Jim Crow laws of the 1890s; and that during Reconstruction, there was considerable economic and political mixing of the races. (Burns collection)

Southwestern States

1. Atkinson, Mary Jourdan. *Creolism & Racism on the Gulf Coast*. Houston: Roots, 1977. 48p. Also published in *Roots* [Houston:

English Dept., Texas Southern University, no. 4 (1977)]. (Dent collection)

2. Creger, Ralph and Carl Creger. *This Is What We Found.* New York: L. Stuart, 1960. 64p. Central High School in Little Rock, Arkansas, reopened in 1959 after a three-year battle between the federal courts and the state government over desegregation. At his father's suggestion, Carl Creger wrote his high-school history paper on the contributions of African Americans and their struggle for equal rights. An expanded version, listing both Carl and Ralph Creger as authors, was published in New York in 1960. (Thompson collection)

3. Wilson, John W. *High John the Conqueror.* New York: Macmillan, 1948. 165p. Review copy from publisher. Story of African American cotton farmers struggling to keep their land during the last years of the Great Depression. Ruby Lee and Cleveland Webster are sharecroppers on property owned by the rich white man, John Cheney, but Cleveland's parents are struggling to hold on to the farm they have owned since the end of slavery. The Webster family land is next on Cheney's list of foreclosures. (Burns collection)

Western States

1. Conot, Robert. *Rivers of Blood, Years of Darkness: The Unforgettable Classic Account of the Watts Riot.* New York: Bantam Books, 1967. 497p. Based on his eyewitness account and extensive interviews, a study of the unrest behind the 1965 riot in Watts, Los Angeles. (Burns collection)

2. Bullock, Paul. *Watts: The Aftermath; An Inside View of the Ghetto, by the People of Watts.* New York: Grove Press, 1970. 285p. Announced in "Ebony Book Shelf," *Ebony*, February 1970, p. 24 Interviews of people who lived through the Watts riot and still live in the community. Content: Watts: Before the Riot; The Riot; After the Riot: Image and Reality; Some Contrasting Impressions of the Community (1966-67); "Leadership" (1967-69); "All Power to the People" (1966-69); Employment and Economics; The Police; Pot

and Pills; The Schools; Welfare; Watts: A View From The Outside. (Thompson collection)

3. Schomburg Center for Research in Black Culture. *The Black West: Pathfinders, Cowpunchers, Homesteadersbysettlers, Oklahoma Land Rush, Buffalo Soldiers, California gold rush, Black Pioneer Women.* New York: Schomburg Center for Research in Black Culture, 1985. 28p. Exhibition held at the Schomburg Center September 16, 1985-January 4, 1986. (Dent collection)

Art and Culture
Authors

1. Hernton, Calvin C. *The Sexual Mountain and Black Women Writers: Adventures in Sex, Literature, and Real Life.* New York: Anchor Press, 1987. 174p. Inscribed by the author to Tom Dent. Content: Who's afraid of Alice Walker?: The Color purple as slave narrative; The sexual mountain and Black women writers; The significance of Ann Petry: the fear of Bigger Thomas and the rage of Lutie Johnson; Black women in the life and work of Langston Hughes: feministic writings of a male poet; Black women poets: the oral narrative tradition; Epilogue. (Dent collection)

2. Hill, Herbert. *Soon One Morning: New Writing by American Negroes, 1940-1962.* New York: Knopf, 1963. 617p. Review copy from publisher. Announced in "Books," *Jet*, November 1, 1962, p. 49; and "Ebony Book Shelf," *Ebony*, August 1963, p. 20. NAACP labor secretary Hill has edited an anthology of fiction, verse and essays by African American writers. (Thompson collection)

3. Williams, Sherley Anne. *Give Birth to Brightness: A Thematic Study in Neo-Black Literature.* New York: Dial, 1972. 252p. Collection of critical essays focusing on the achievements of twentieth-century African American writers. Offers thematic analyses of their work and of black archetypes appearing in their fiction. Partial content include: The heroic tradition in Black Americana; Rebel and streetman in Black literature; The limitations of a middle-class "hero"; The limited solution of revolution; The Black musician: the

Black hero as law breaker; The streetman: the Black hero as light bearer; The demands of Blackness on contemporary critics. (Burns collection)

Jazz Music

1. Stewart, Charles and Paul Carter Harrison. *Chuck Stewart's Jazz Files.* Boston: Little, Brown, 1985. 144p. An introduction to various jazz musicians that the New York photographer has come to know throughout a period of three decades, from Duke Ellington to David Murray. (Dent collection)

2. Goffin, Robert. *Jazz, From the Congo to the Metropolitan.* Garden City, NY: Doubleday, Doran & Co., 1944. 254p. Burns ownership inscription. Includes Burns' book review from the *Chicago Defender* national edition ("Books," February 5, 1944, p. 13). Annotations in the form of vertical line markings in margins. Translated from the French by Walter Schaap and Leonard G. Feather. From African rhythms to international influences, it traces the emergence of the American contribution to music, with emphasis on the leaders, the bands, white as well as African American. (Burns collection)

3. Baldwin, James. *Another Country.* New York: Dial Press, 1962. 436p. Inscribed by the author to Thompson. Reviewed in "Book of the Week," *Jet*, July 5, 1962, p. 48. Deals with race relationships and homosexuality. Story of the suicide of Harlem jazz musician Rufus Scott and the friends who search for an understanding of his life and death, discovering uncomfortable truths about themselves along the way. (Thompson collection)

Athletes

1. Scott, Neil. *Joe Louis: Picture Story of His Life.* New York: Greenberg, 1947. 126p. Based on research and first-hand interviews, presents Louis and his impact on sports and country. At a time when the boxing ring was the only venue where black and white

could meet on equal terms, Louis embodied African American hopes for dignity and equality. (Burns collection)

2. Robinson, Jackie. *My Own Story, as Told to Wendell Smith.* New York: Greenberg, 1948. 170p. Foreword by Branch Rickey. Featured in "My Own Story," *Ebony*, June 1948, pp. 19-24. About the first black baseball player to integrate the major leagues. (Thompson collection)

3. Hoberman, John M. *Darwin's Athletes: How Sport has Damaged Black America and Preserved the Myth of Race.* Boston: Houghton Mifflin Co., 1997. 341p. Content: The African-American sports fixation; Jackie Robinson's sad song: the resegregation of American sport; Joe Louis meets Albert Einstein: the athleticizing of the black mind; The suppression of the black male action figure; "Writin' is fightin'": sport and the black intellectuals; Wonders out of Africa; The world of colonial sport; The new multiracial world order; The fastest white man in the world; Imagining the black organism; The Negro as a defective type; African-American responses to racial biology; Black "hardiness" and the origins of medical racism; Theories of racial athletic aptitude; Athleticizing the black criminal; The fear of racial biology. (Dent collection)

Women

1. Williams, Ora. *American Black Women in the Arts and Sciences: A Bibliographic Survey.* Metuchen, NJ: Scarecrow Press, 1973. 141p. An expanded and revised version of an article published in the *CLA Journal* (March 1972), vol. 15, no. 3, pp. 354-377. Includes literature, culinary arts, musical conductors, college presidents among other fields. (Burns collection)

2. Brown, Helen Gurley. *Sex and the Single Girl.* New York: B. Geiss Associates, dist. by Random House, 1962. 267p. Announced in "Ebony Book Shelf," *Ebony*, February 1963, p 21. There also was an announcement in *Jet* magazine about band leader Count Basie's role as a night club owner in the film version of Helen Gurley Brown's best seller (*Jet*, October 31, 1963, p. 58). Nearly a year

later Helen Gurley Brown is quoted as saying "Just because more women are sleeping with more men and enjoying it doesn't mean that society has decayed" in "Words of the Week," *Jet*, November 27, 1964, p. 30. (Thompson collection)

3. *Six Women's Slave Narratives.* New York: Oxford University Press, 1989. 328p. With an introduction by William L. Andrews. Content: The history of Mary Prince, West Indian slave originally edited by Thomas Pringle; Memoir of old Elizabeth, a coloured woman; The story of Mattie J. Jackson written and arranged by L. S. Thompson; From the darkness cometh the light or struggles for freedom by Lucy A. Delaney; A slave girl's story by Kate Drumgoold; Memories of childhood's slavery days by Annie L. Burton. (Dent collection)

Political Affairs
Presidents

1. Edsall, Thomas Byrne and Mary D. Edsall. *Chain Reaction: The Impact of Race, Rights, and Taxes on American Politics.* New York: Norton, 1991. 339p. Content: Building a top-down coalition; A pivotal year; After 1964: the fraying consensus; The Nixon years; The conservative ascendance; The tax revolt; Race, rights, and party choice; A conservative policy majority; The Reagan attack on race liberalism; Coded language: "groups,, "taxes," "big government," and "special interests"; White suburbs and a divided black community; The stakes. (Dent collection; also copy in the Thompson collection)

2. Saunders, Doris E. *The Kennedy Years and the Negro, a Photographic Record.* Chicago: Johnson Pub. Co., 1964. 143p. An illustrated photographic record with an introduction by Associate White House Press Secretary, and first black to hold such a post, Andrew T. Hatcher. (Burns collection)

3. Truman, Margaret. *Harry S. Truman.* New York: Morrow, 1973. 602p. His daughter paints an in-depth portrait of the politician

from Missouri who, in the midst of World War II, succeeded Franklin D. Roosevelt as President of the United States. (Thompson collection)

Politics and Government

1. Clayton, Ed. *The Negro Politician, His Success and Failure*. Chicago: Johnson Pub. Co., 1964. 213p. Announced in "Backstage," *Ebony*, October 1962, p. 22. Former *Jet* magazine editor Edward T. Clayton chronicles black political life in the United States since the Emancipation Proclamation with special attention to the 20 years prior to the works publication. (Thompson collection)

2. Morrison, Minion K. C. *Black Political Mobilization: Leadership, Power, and Mass Behavior*. Albany, NY: State University of New York Press, 1987. 303p. Annotated. Content: The American political system and mobilization politics; Black and white in the southern regional context; Neo-populism in Bolton; Heroine in Mayersville; Agrarian townsman in Tchula; The electorates: politics, economics and ideology; The political economy of rural Black-American mobilization. (Dent collection)

3. Wilson, James Q. *Negro Politics: The Search for Leadership*. Glencoe, IL: Free Press, 1960. 242p. Data collected from interviews with black leaders in Chicago, Detroit, New York, and Los Angeles. Focuses primarily on the political and civic life of Chicago's black community. Partial content include: Part I: The Organization of Negro Political Life; Part II: The Organization of Negro Civic Life; Part III: The Character of Negro Public Life. (Burns collection)

Human Rights
Civil Rights

1. Isaacs, Harold R. *The New World of Negro Americans: A Study from the Center for International Studies, Massachusetts Institute of Technology*. New York: John Day Co, 1963. 366p. Announced in "Ebony Book Shelf," *Ebony*, August 1963, p. 20. Based on 107

interviews with African Americans including many living in Africa. Purpose is to show how the end of world white supremacy is forcing the end of the white supremacy system here, and how these changes affect the lives and thinking of American blacks. (Thompson collection)

2. Garrow, David J. *Protest at Selma: Martin Luther King, Jr., and the Voting Rights Act of 1965*. New Haven, CT: Yale University Press, 1978. 346p. Revision of the author's senior honors thesis (Wesleyan University, 1973). Annotated. Content: Introduction: voting rights and protest; Black voters and the federal voting rights enforcement effort in the South, 1940-1964; Selma and the Voting Rights Act: commencement and climax; Selma and the Voting Rights Act: crisis and denouement; Reactions and responses: Selma, Birmingham, and civil rights legislation; Congressmen, constituents, and the news media; Enforcement and effects: the Voting Rights Act and black political participation in the South, 1965-1976; The strategy of protest and the SCLC at Selma. (Dent collection)

3. Williams, Robert F. *Negroes with Guns*. New York: Manzani & Munsell, 1962. 128p. About a southern black community's struggle to arm itself in self-defense against the Ku Klux Klan and other racist groups. Content includes Williams' interview with Marc Schleifer, his articles and editorials from the Crusader newsletter, an interview with John Schultz first published in *Studies on the Left*, and the articles "Hate is always tragic" and "The social organization of non-violence" by M. L. King, Jr.; and "The resistant spirit" by T. Nelson. (Burns collection)

Insurrections

1. Bartlett, Vernon. *Struggle for Africa*. New York: F. A. Praeger, 1953. 246p. Former *London Times* newspaper correspondent's surveys Africa. Covers South African Boer nationalism and racial intolerance, whites and blacks working towards a stable society in Belgium Congo, Nigeria and the Gold Coast where black autonomy was nearly realized, religious and political turbulence in

Morocco, Algeria and Tunisia, and Kenya's Mau Mau insurrection. (Thompson collection)

2. Lofton, John. *Denmark Vesey's Revolt: The Slave Plot that Lit a Fuse to Fort Sumter.* Kent, OH: Kent State University Press, 1983. 294p. Updated ed. of *Insurrection in South Carolina* (1964). Annotated. Traces the history of the attempted revolt and its repercussions, including the passage of the Negro Seaman Act by the South Carolina Legislature, the first time the state usurped power from the federal government. (Dent collection)

3. Quarles, Benjamin. *Blacks on John Brown.* Urbana: University of Illinois Press, 1972. 164p. Brings together writings on John Brown including personal letters, eulogies, sermons, essays, and newspaper articles. (Burns collection)

Nationalism

1. Benson, Mary. *The African Patriots, the Story of the African National Congress of South Africa.* London: Faber and Faber, 1963. 310p. Handwritten notes written on inserts. This book is a history of the African National Congress and many of the battles it experienced. Partial content include: 1910-1912: The foundation; 1918-1924: 1943-1944: The Youth League; 1949-1951: The programme of action; 1955-1956: Women under way. (Thompson collection)

2. Biko, Steve. *Black Consciousness in South Africa.* Edited by Millard W. Arnold. New York: Random House, 1978. 298p. Biko's testimony at the trial of his nine colleagues in the Black Consciousness movement reveals his positions on political freedom, revolution, racism, and the need for the cultural and psychological liberation of South Africa's blacks. Content: I write what I like: fear, an important determinant in South African politics by Frank Talk (a.k.a. Steve Biko); The inquest into the death of Stephen Bantu Biko: a report to the Lawyers' Committee for Civil Rights Under Law by Dean Louis H. Pollak. (Dent Collection)

3. Orizu, Nwafor, Sir. *Without Bitterness; Western Nations in Post-War*

Africa. New York: Creative Age Press, 1944. 395p. Review copy from publisher. Annotations in the form of vertical line markings in margins. A commentary on African and Western ways of life, a personal moral and political philosophy, and a program for the emancipation of Nigeria. (Burns collection)

Revolutions

1. Fanon, Frantz. *The wretched of the earth*. New York: Grove Press, 1963. 316p. Translation of *Damnés de la terre* by Constance Farrington. Psychological analysis of decolonization. An effect of imperialism is that national consciousness degenerates in to petty identity politics when the middle class (educated by the colonial power) seeks its own benefit over that of the masses. (Burns collection; copy of 1996 edition in the Dent collection)

2. James, C. L. R. *The Black Jacobins: Toussaint L'Ouverture and the San Domingo Revolution*. New York: Vintage Books, 1963. 426p. 2nd ed., rev. Annotated by Dent. Describes the successful slave revolt of 1791 and establishment of Haiti as an independent nation. (Dent collection)

3. Wright, Richard. *Black Power: A Record of Reactions in a Land of Pathos*. New York: Harper, 1954. 358p. Annotations in the form of horizontal line markings. Inscribed by Adeline Pynchon to Thompson: "For Era Bell Thompson with love from her friend." Richard Wright visits Accra, as guest of the leader. Sees the results of those forces of geography that made the country rich in raw materials and prey to British imperialism. Reports on the revolution of Africa's Gold Coast. (Thompson collection)

International Affairs
Foreign Relations

1. Skinner, Elliott P. *African Americans and U.S. Policy toward Africa, 1850-1924: in Defense of Black Nationality*. Washington, DC: Howard University Press, 1992. 555p. Annotated. (Dent collection)

2. Kugelmass, J. Alvin. *Ralph J. Bunche: Fighter for Peace*. New York: Messner, 1952. 174p. Reviewed in "Book of the Week," *Jet*, November 13, 1952, p. 46. Retells familiar story of Bunche's childhood, his education and UCLA and Harvard, his teaching career, his projection into the world spotlight as a UN mediator in Palestine, and a Nobel Peace Prize winner in 1950. (Thompson collection; copy also in the Burns collection)

3. Maisel, Albert Q. *Africa, Facts and Forecasts*. New York: Duell, Sloan and Pearce, 1943. 307p. Annotations in the form of vertical line markings in margins. Includes Aug. 6, 1973 invoice from Time-Life Books, 541 North Fairbanks Court, Chicago, IL 60611. With a series of photographic maps. Written to provide information to those who know little about Africa and to show its importance in the international conflict, its use in the invasion of Europe. (Burns collection)

Colonialism

1. Du Bois, W. E. B. *Color and Democracy: colonies and peace*. New York: Harcourt, Brace & Co., 1945. 143p. Review copy from publisher. Content: Dumbarton Oaks; The disenfranchised colonies; The unfree peoples; Democracy and color; Peace and colonies; The riddle of Russia; Missions and mandates. (Burns collection)

2. Lewis, David L. *The Race to Fashoda: European Colonialism and African Resistance in the Scramble for Africa*. New York: Weidenfeld & Nicolson, 1987. 304p. Annotated. The last three decades of the 19th century saw an effort by the major European powers to colonize the interior of the African continent. Draws from the archives of African states, political correspondence, and memoirs. Focuses on the Nile Valley region in North Africa. The last three decades of the 19th century saw an effort by the major European powers to colonize the interior of the African continent. (Dent collection)

3. Ruark, Robert Chester. *Something of Value*. Garden City, NY: Doubleday, 1955. 566p. Peter McKenzie is a professional hunter in colonial Kenya whose idyllic life is disrupted by the Mau Mau

insurrection of the 1950s, an uprising that was confined almost exclusively to the Kikuyu. (Thompson collection)

Missions and Missionaries

1. Achebe, Chinua. *Things Fall Apart.* New York: Fawcett Crest Books, 1969. 192p. Includes a glossary of Igbo words and phrases on page 192. Annotations in the form of horizontal line markings throughout chapters 18, 20-22. Intertwining stories about Okonkwo, a man from an Igbo village in Nigeria. The first of these stories traces Okonkwo's fall from grace with the tribal world in which he lives. The second story concerns the clash of cultures and the destruction of Okonkwo's world through the arrival of European missionaries. (Dent collection; also copy in the Burns collection)

2. Hagedorn, Hermann. *Prophet in the Wilderness: The Story of Albert Schweitzer.* New York: Macmillan Co., 1947. 221p. Review copy from publisher. Biography of Albert Schweitzer, holder of doctorates in medicine, theology, philosophy, and music. As a medical missionary in Africa, urges faith and reverence for life. (Burns collection)

3. Wright, Charlotte Crogman. *Beneath the Southern Cross: The Story of an American Bishop's Wife in South Africa.* New York: Exposition Press, 1955. 184p. (Thompson collection)

Race Relations
Armed Forces

1. Gropman, Alan L. *The Air Force Integrates, 1945-1964.* Washington, DC: Office of Air Force History, 1978. 384p. Study based on unpublished records that show how Air Force integration proceeded from a 1945 protest at Freeman Field, Indiana through the administrations of Presidents Truman and Kennedy. (Burns collection)

2. Greene, Robert Ewell. *Black Defenders of America, 1775-1973.* Chicago: Johnson Pub. Co., 1974. 416p. Mentioned as newly published book in "The Old Soldier Who Wouldn't Surrender," *Ebony,* November, 1974, p. 90. African American's part in defending America from the Revolutionary War to the Vietnam crisis is revealed in photographs and biographical sketches. (Thompson collection)

3. Taylor, Susie King. *A Black Woman's Civil War Memoirs: Reminiscences of My Life in Camp with the 33rd U.S. Colored Troops, Late 1st South Carolina Volunteers.* New York: M. Wiener Pub.; dist. by the Talman Co., 1988. 154p. Originally published in 1902 as *Reminiscences of My Life in Camp with the 33d United States Colored Troops, Late 1st S.C. Volunteers.* Annotated. Content: A brief sketch of my ancestors; My childhood; On St. Simon's Island, 1862; Camp Saxton--proclamation and barbecue, 1863; Military expeditions, and life in camp; On Morris and other islands; Cast away; A flag of truce; Capture of Charleston; Mustered out; After the war; The Women's Relief Corps; Thoughts on present conditions; A visit to Louisiana. (Dent collection)

Interracial Sex
(and the associated terms such as miscegenation, biracial identity, interracial dating, etc.)

1. Barron, Milton Leon. *People Who Intermarry.* Syracuse, NY: Syracuse University Press, 1946. 389p. Burns ownership inscription. (Burns collection)

2. Murray, Pauli. *Proud Shoes: The Story of an American Family.* New York: Harper, 1956. 276p. An African American lawyer, civil rights activist, and Episcopal priest comes to terms with her origins as she tells of the miscegenation, slavery, and struggles that are integral parts of her family's past. History of a family blended from slaves, free blacks, white slaveowners, Cherokee Indians, and others. (Thompson collection)

3. Walker, Margaret. *Jubilee.* New York: Bantam Books, 1967. 416p. First published in 1966 by Houghton Mifflin. Novel about the for-

tunes of a mulatto girl, as a slave during the Civil War and then as a woman freed by the Emancipation Proclamation. (Dent collection)

Lynching

1. Schwartz, Irving. *Every Man His Sword*. Garden City, NY: Doubleday, 1951. 307p. Review copy from publisher. Three white men tie a black man to the rear bumper of a car and drag him through the streets of a small southern town until he is dead. All three white men are killed by a Jewish man in retaliation. (Burns collection)

2. Smead, Howard. *Blood Justice: The Lynching of Mack Charles Parker*. New York: Oxford University Press, 1986. 248p. (Dent collection)

3. Smith, Lillian Eugenia. *Strange Fruit: A Novel*. New York: Harcourt, Brace & World, 1944. 250p. Bookplate of Thompson. Prelude and aftermath of a lynching in Georgia, depicting the South's unsolved racial problem. With a title taken from a Billie Holiday song about a lynching, the novel sparked immediate controversy and tempted the public enough to make it the years's No. 1 fiction best-seller. (Thompson collection; also a copy in the Burns collection)

Passing (identity)

1. White, W. L. *Lost Boundaries*. New York: Harcourt Brace, 1947. 83p. Review copy from publisher. Story of a New England family who, upon finding out about their black ancestry, were confronted with the decision whether to maintain their white "front" or publicly accept their black past. (Burns collection)

2. Lewis, Sinclair. *Kingsblood Royal*. New York: Random House, 1947. 348p. Annual award from *Ebony*, June 1947, for best book promoting interracial understanding. The protagonist, Neil Kingsblood, discovers that he has black ancestry and thus by state law is black. (Thompson collection)

3. Wright, Arthur. *Color Me White: The Autobiography of a Black Dancer Who Turned White*. Smithtown, NY: Exposition Press, 1980. 372p. A November 1978 article in *Ebony* magazine about Wright describes his experiences with vitiligo and his decision to undergo a complete depigmentation of his skin in order to live a normal life. (Dent collection)

Slavery

1. Marx, Karl, Frederick Engels and Richard Enmale. *Civil war in the United States*. New York: International Publishers, 1937. 325p. Burns ownership inscription. Contains 42 articles from the New York *Daily Tribune* and the Vienna*Presse*, and extracts from 61 letters between Marx and Engels. Marx recognized that slavery had divided the American republic into two opposing social systems and that in the final outcome the very existence of slavery was at stake. (Burns collection)

2. Price, Richard. *Maroon Societies: Rebel Slave Communities in the Americas*. Garden City, NY: Anchor Press, 1973. 429p. Annotated. Historical accounts, written by slaves and slavers, anthropological studies, and researched papers which examine maroon societies over the centuries. (Dent collection)

3. Montejo, Esteban. *The Autobiography of a Runaway Slave*. New York: Pantheon Books, 1968. 223p. Edited by Miguel Barnet. Translation of *Biografia de un Cimarron* by Jocasta Innes. Reviewed in "Recent and Useful Texts on Afro-American Life and History," *Negro Digest*, February 1969, p. 76-78. Autobiography of 108 year old black Cuban divided into 3 parts: Slavery, Abolition, War of Independence. (Thompson collection)

Soldiers

1. Killens, John Oliver. *And Then We Heard the Thunder*. New York: Knopf, 1963. 485p. Handwritten notes on insert. Announced in "Ebony Book Shelf," *Ebony*, April 1963, p. 21. "Take one Negro

sergeant, assign him a white Southern captain and a Jewish lieutenant, then add three women, all of them in love with him and you have this lusty story told by Solly Saunders, the sargent." (Thompson collection)

2. Terry, Wallace. *Bloods: An Oral History of the Vietnam War*. New York: Random House, 1984. 311p. Annotated. Reviewed by Dent (Thomas Covington Dent Papers. Series 2: Box 39. Folder 22). Features twenty black men who discuss their Vietnam War experiences in their own words. (Dent collection)

3. White, Walter Francis. *A Rising Wind: A Report on the Negro Soldier in the European Theatre of War*. Garden City, NY: Doubleday, Doran & Co., 1945. 155p. Review copy from publisher. Firsthand report by former journalist and executive secretary of the National Association for the Advancement of Colored People about status of blacks in war theatres in England, Italy and Africa. (Burns collection)

World War II

1. Christian, Marcus Bruce. *The Common Peoples' Manifesto of World War II*. New Orleans: Les Cenelles Society of Arts & Letters, 1948. 28p. Written in 1943, Christian published it on his own press. Named one of the outstanding black books of 1948 earning the National Association for the Advancement of Colored People's Arthur Spingarn Award. Content: Proem: Men on horseback; The common peoples' manifesto, a poem written in five parts; Apologia: The ballad of rebellious men. (Thompson collection)

2. Mandelbaum, David G. *Soldier Groups and Negro Soldiers*. Berkeley: University of California Press, 1952. 142p. Review copy from publisher. Contains two essays, the second of which deals with the racially integrated vs. the racially segregated military unit. Mandelbaum advocates the latter. Partial content includes: Negroes in the Army before World War II, World War II experience; The Navy: from exclusion to integration; The Air Force: toward the abandonment of segregation; The Army: toward modification of segrega-

tion; Results of new Army policy; and Korean combat. (Burns collection)

3. Potter, Lou, with William Miles and Nina Rosenblum. *Liberators: Fighting on Two Fronts in World War II*. New York: Harcourt Brace Jovanovich, 1992. 303p. A companion book to the television documentary under the same title presented by Public Broadcasting System as part of its "American experience" series, Veterans Day, 1992. (Dent collection)

Social Conditions
Discrimination

1. Conrad, Earl. *Jim Crow America*. New York: Duell, Sloan and Pearce, 1947. 237p. Inscribed by the author to Burns. Annotations in the form of vertical line markings in margins. White journalist and former head of the New York office of the *Chicago Defender* discusses economic conditions, the resurgence of black literature, rural-urban migration, the white press, housing segregation, history, African heritage, black organizations and leadership. (Burns collection)

2. Lubell, Samuel. *White and Black: Test of a Nation*. New York: Harper & Row, 1964. 210p. Review copy from publisher. Reviewed in "Ebony Book Shelf," *Ebony*, October 1964, p. 24. Reviews country's handling of racial conflict during the 100 years since emancipation. Concludes that the North should concentrate on abolishing discrimination in housing and the South on abolishing public discrimination against blacks and integrating the schools. (Thompson collection)

3. Shipler, David K. *A Country of Strangers: Blacks and Whites in America*. New York: Knopf, 1997. 607p. Review copy; uncorrected proof. Annotated. Reviewed by Dent (Thomas Covington Dent Papers. Series 2: Box 39. Folder 28). Content: Introduction: The Color Line; Pt. 1: Origins. 1. Integration: Together and Separate. 2. Mixing: The Stranger Within. 3. Memory: The Echoes of History; Pt. 2: Images. 4. Body: Dark Against the Sky. 5. Mind: Through a

Glass, Darkly. 6. Morality: Black Heat, White Cold. 7. Violence: The Mirror of Harm. 8. Power: The Natural Order; Pt. 3: Choices. 9. Decoding Racism. 10. Acting Affirmatively. 11. Breaking the Silence. 12. A Country of Strangers. (Dent collection)

Economic Conditions

1. Pierce, Joseph A. *Negro Business and Business Education*. Westport, CT: Greenwood Press, 1971. 338p. Burns ownership inscription. Originally published as Atlanta University Publications, no. 24 (Harper, 1947). Author believes that black businesses must cooperate through the formation of purchasing and trade associations, and integration through partnerships with white people. (Burns collection)

2. Rowan, Carl T. *Just Between Us Blacks*. New York: Random House, 1974. 202p. Inscribed by Gwen Ifill to Thompson. Announced in "Books," *Jet*, December 26, 1974, p. 55. Makes cutting attacks on white racism and criticizes blacks who fail to use the liberties and opportunities already gained. (Thompson collection)

3. Rodney, Walter. *How Europe Underdeveloped Africa*. Washington: Howard University Press, 1974. 288p. Content: Chapter One. Some Questions on Development. Chapter Two. How Africa Developed Before the Coming of the Europeans up to the 15th Century. Chapter Three. Africa's Contribution to European Capitalist Development - the Pre-Colonial Period. Chapter Four. Europe and the Roots of African Underdevelopment - to 1885. Chapter Five. Africa's Contribution to the Capitalist Development of Europe - the Colonial Period. Chapter Six. Colonialism as a System for Underdeveloping Africa. (Dent collection)

Education

1. Ginzberg, Eli. The Negro potential. New York: Columbia University Press, 1956. 144p. Published after a 5 year study at Columbia University. Concludes that the South will have to give up the

luxury of maintaining segregation in the workplace if it continues to lose its most competent and best trained black workers. (Thompson collection)

2. Oakes, Jeannie. *Keeping Track: How Schools Structure Inequality*. New Haven, CT: Yale University Press, 1985. 231p. Annotated. Examines how grouping students in classes based on ability reveals the class and racial inequalities of American society and helps perpetuate those equalities. (Dent collecton)

3. Woodson, Carter Godwin. *Mis-education of the Negro*. Washington, DC: Associated Publishers, 1969. 215p. Stamped Board of Education, City of Chicago; inscribed Eva S. Butler. (Burns collection; also a copy in the Dent collection)

Housing

1. Weaver, Robert C. *Negro Ghetto*. New York: Harcourt, Brace, 1948. 404p. Review copy from publisher. Executive director of the mayor's committee on race relations in Chicago, having prepared a brief to help win the Supreme Court decision against racial covenants, discusses residential segregation and public housing projects in the North. (Burns collection)

2. Huddleston, Trevor. *Naught for Your Comfort*. Garden City, NY: Doubleday, 1956. 253p. An Anglican missionary and educator who lived for 12 years in South Africa protests slums, overcrowding in urban areas, and racial segregation in that country. (Thompson collection)

3. Jacobs, Jane. *The Death and Life of Great American Cities*. New York: Vintage Books, 1992. 458p. Originally published in 1961 by Random House. Partial content: Forces of decline and regeneration: The self-destruction of diversity: The curse of border vacuums; Unslumming and slumming. Subsidizing dwellings; Salvaging projects; Governing and planning districts; The kind of problem a city is. (Dent collection)

Domestic Violence/Sexual Abuse

1. Angelou, Maya. *I Know Why the Caged Bird Sings*. New York: Random House, 1969. 281p. About the early years of the African American writer and poet. Period covered is from 3 to 17 years-old, describing abandonment, rape, and racial intolerance. Biography ends when Maya becomes a mother at the age of 17. (Thompson collection)

2. Caldwell, Erskine. *Place Called Estherville*. New York: New American Library, 1952. 158p. About the struggles of a black brother and sister in their attempt to survive the racism and perverse sexuality of their brutal Southern employers. (Burns collection)

3. Walker, Alice. *The Color Purple: A Novel*. New York: Harcourt Brace Jovanovich, 1982. 245p. Set in the period between the world wars, this novel tells of two sisters, their trials, and their survival. (Dent collection)

Segregation

1. Feagin, Joe R. and Melvin P. Sikes. *Living With Racism: The Black Middle-Class Experience*. Boston: Beacon Press, 1994. 398p. Content: The continuing significance of racism; Navigating public places; Seeking a good education; Navigating the middle-class workplace; Building a business; Seeking a good home and neighborhood; Contending with everyday discrimination; Changing the color line: the future of U.S. racism. (Dent collection)

2. King, Martin Luther, Jr. *Stride Toward Freedom*. New York: Harper, 1958. 230p. Announced in "Books," *Jet*, September 11, 1958, p. 41. A chronicle of the experiences of the cleric and his followers during the successful Montgomery bus boycott, has been called "must" reading by Mrs. Eleanor Roosevelt. (Thompson collection)

3. Smith, Lillian Eugenia. *Killers of the Dream*. New York: Norton, 1949. 256p. Annotations in the form of vertical line markings in

margins. Cites the evils of segregation for both white and black people and gives the history of race relations from pre-Civil War days. (Burns collection)

Social Classes

1. Packard, Vance. *The Status Seekers: An Exploration of Class Behavior in America and the Hidden Barriers That Affect You, Your Community, Your Future.* New York: D. McKay Co., 1959. 376p. Annotations in the form of horizontal line markings. Mentioned in editorial "The Negro Status Seeker" *Ebony*, January 1960, p. 96. "Members of ethnic groups who successfully pass the horizontal tests of prestige, says Vance Packard in his much-discussed book, …face the vertical barriers of race and religion. That puts the Negro squarely at the bottom of a two-dimensional class system in a double standard society of a basically bi-racial world. He not only has the exhausting task of catching up with the white Joneses, but also keeping up with the black Jacksons." (Thompson collection)

2. Warner, W. Lloyd, Robert J. Havighurst and Martin B. Loeb. *Who Shall Be Educated?: The Challenge of Unequal Opportunities.* New York: Harper & Bros., 1944. 190p. Burns ownership inscription. Annotations in the form of vertical line markings in margins. Holds that school system is a social institution that perpetuates the existing social structure while at the same time providing opportunity for a limited amount of social mobility. (Burns collection)

3. Rodney, Walter. *A History of the Guyanese Working People, 1881-1905.* Baltimore, MD: Johns Hopkins University Press, 1981. 282p. Content:1. Internal and external constraints on the development of the working people; 2. The evolution of the plantation labor force in the nineteenth century; 3. Crisis and creativity in the small-farming sectors; 4. Socioeconomic differentiation: on the coast and in the hinterland; 5. The politics of the middle classes and the masses, 1880-1892; 6. Resistance and accommodation; 7. Race as a contradiction among the working people; 8. The 1905 riots (Dent collection)

Social Conditions

1. Boykin, Keith. *One More River to Cross: Black and Gay in America*. New York: Anchor Books/Doubleday, 1998. 272p. Originally published in 1996. Content: In search of home; Are Blacks and gays the same?; Black and gay in America; Bearing witness: faith in the lives of Black lesbians and gays; Black homophobia; Gay racism; Deja Vu: the common language of racism and homophobia; One more river to cross. (Dent collection)

2. Frazier, E. Franklin. *Negro Family in the United States*. Revised and abridged ed. New York: Dryden Press, 1948. 374p. Review copy from publisher. Beginning with colonial-era slavery, extending through the years of slavery and emancipation, to the impact of Jim Crow and migrations to both southern and northern cities in the twentieth century. Insisted that the characteristics of the family were shaped not by race, but by social conditions. (Burns collection)

3. Kardiner, Abram and Lionel Ovesey. *The Mark of Oppression: Explorations in the Personality of the American Negro*. Cleveland, OH: World Pub. Co., 1962. 396p. A compilation of psychoanalytic case histories based on information given by 25 resident of Harlem. Arrives at sweeping conclusion that no African American can escape the psychological scars of racial discrimination. (Thompson collection; copy also in the Burns collection)

Social Life and Customs
Religion

1. Landes, Ruth. *The City of Women*. New York: Macmillan, 1947. 248p. Anthropologist Landes' study is about Afro-Brazilian candomble, a woman-centered spirit possession religion evolved by West African slaves in colonial plantation societies. (Burns collection)

2. Jenkins, Ulysses Duke. *Ancient African Religion and the African-American Church*. Jacksonville, NC: Flame International, 1978.

158p. Presentation copy inscribed "To Era Bell on her Birthday. Many happy, happy! With love, Louise 1979." (Thompson collection)

3. Métraux, Alfred. *Voodoo in Haiti*. New York: Schocken Books, 1972. 400p. Originally published in French as *Le Vaudou Haïtien* (Gallimard, 1958). Translated by Hugo Charteris. Content: Origins and history of the voodoo cults; The social framework of voodoo; Voodoo clergy and cult-groups; The sanctuaries; Gods and spirits in Haitian voodoo; The power of the loa; The voodoo pantheon; Possession; Epiphany of the gods; Dreams; The cult of twins; Animist beliefs; Ritual; The ritual salutations; The flag parade; Invocation formulae; The libations; Orientation rites; Material representations of divinity; The sacrifice; Offerings; Music and dance; Initiation rites in Haitian voodoo; Mystical marriage in voodoo; The conjuring up of loa; The feast of yams; Voodoo Christmas in Haiti; The cult of the dead; Magic and sorcery; The societies of sorcerers; White magic; Ordeals; Divination; Voodoo and Christianity. (Dent collection)

Rural-Urban Migration

1. Attaway, William. *Blood on the Forge: A Novel*. New York: Popular Library, 1953. Three African-American brothers leave their home as sharecroppers in Kentucky to work in the steel mills of Pittsburgh prior to World War One, encountering the harsh realities of industrialization. (Burns collection)

2. Drake, St. Clair and Horace R. Cayton. *Black Metropolis: A Study of Negro Life in a Northern City*. New York: Harper & Row, 1962. 2 vols. An historical and sociological account of the people of Chicago's South Side. Offers an analysis of rural-urban migration, settlement, community structure, and black-white race relations in the early part of the twentieth century. (Thompson collection; also 1945 edition in Burns; and 2-vol. 1970 set is in the Dent collection)

3. Walls, Dwayne E. *The Chickenbone Special*. New York: Harcourt

Brace Jovanovich, 1971. 233p. Annotated. Chronicles the experiences of rural Southerners who have left their homes in search of new opportunities and new hope in the North. (Dent collection)

Social Life and Customs

1. Hughes, Langston. *The Ways of White Folks*. New York: Knopf, 1947. 248p. Inscribed by the author to Thompson. Content: Cora unashamed; Slave on the block; Home; Passing; A good job gone; Rejuvenation through joy; The blues I'm playing; Red-headed baby; Poor little black fellow; Little dog; Berry; Mother and child; One Christmas Eve; Father and son. (Thompson collection)

2. Ojike, Mbonu. *My Africa*. New York: John Day Co., 1946. 350p. Annotations in the form of vertical line markings in margins. Introduction by Pearl Buck. Concerned chiefly with Nigeria (rural Nigerian life, history, demography, resources, culture, trade, political and economic conditions, and British colonialism). (Burns collection)

3. Herskovits, Melville J. *The Myth of the Negro Past*. Boston: Beacon Press, 1958. 368p. Annotated. Debunks the myth that black Americans have no cultural past. Partial content include: The Significance of Africanisms; The African Cultural Heritage; Enslavement and the Reaction to Slave Status; The Contemporary Scene: Africanisms in Secular Life; The Contemporary Scene: Africanisms in Religious Life; The Contemporary Scene: Language and the Arts. (Dent collection)

Social Movements
Abolitionists

1. Gilbert, Olive and Sojourner Truth. *Narrative of Sojourner Truth: A Bondswoman of Olden Time: Emancipated by the New York Legislature in the Early Part of the Present Century: With a History of Her Labors and Correspondence Drawn from Her Book of Life*. Chicago: Johnson Pub. Co., 1970. 240p. Originally published Boston by F.

W. Titus in 1875. Autobiography of the pioneer for racial and sexual equality discusses her years as a slave in upstate New York and describes the spiritual revelations that turned her into an abolitionist. (Thompson collection)

2. Quarles, Benjamin. *Blacks on John Brown*. Urbana: University of Illinois Press, 1972. 164p. Annotated. (Dent collection)

3. Wolf, Hazel Catherine. *On Freedom's Altar: The Martyr Complex in the Abolition Movement*. Madison: University of Wisconsin Press, 1952. 195p. Burns ownership inscription. Summarizes careers of three abolitionists who gave their lives espousing emancipationist doctrines between the early 18th century and Civil War: Elijah Lovejoy, Charles Turner Torrey, and John Brown. Also sketches experiences of numerous other abolitionists. (Burns collection)

Antislavery Movements

1. Blackett, R. J. M. *Building an Antislavery Wall: Black Americans in the Atlantic Abolitionist Movement, 1830-1860*. Baton Rouge: Louisiana State University Press, 1983. 237p. Examines the efforts of black Americans in England to advance the cause of their own freedom. (Dent collection)

2. Still, William. *The Underground Railroad: A Record of Facts, Authentic Narratives, Letters, &c. Narrating the Hardships Hair-Breadth Escapes and Death Struggles of the Slaves in Their Efforts for Freedom, as Related by Themselves and Others, or Witnessed by the Author; Together with Sketches of Some of the Largest Stockholders, and Most Liberal Aiders and Advisers of the Road*. Chicago: Johnson Pub. Co., 1970. 1812p. Originally published in 1872 by Porter & Coates. Announced in "Books," *Jet*, July 16, 1970, p.45 as one of six books inaugurating the *Ebony Classics* series. (Thompson collection)

3. Thomas, Benjamin Platt. *Theodore Weld: Crusader for Freedom*. New Brunswick, NJ: Rutgers University Press, 1950. 307p. Burns ownership inscription. Theodore Dwight Weld (1803-1895), a prominent abolitionist and reformer. Weld married Angelina Grimke,

one of a pair of South Carolina sisters who had became antislavery and women's rights activists. (Burns collection)

Civil Rights

1. Beifuss, Joan Turner. *At the River I Stand: Memphis, the 1968 Strike, and Martin Luther King.* Memphis: B & W Books, 1985. 370p. 110. Inscribed by author. Annotated. Beifuss' award-winning book is based on oral histories in the University of Memphis Sanitation Strike Collection. Explains the most far-reaching and volatile event in Memphis history. (Dent collection)

2. Owens, Jesse and Paul G. Niemark. *Blackthink: My Life as Black Man and White Man.* New York: Morrow, 1970. 215p. Annotations in the form of horizontal line markings. Review copy from publisher. Reviewed by Era Bell Thompson in *Chicago Sun-Times* [Era Bell Thompson Papers. Box 7. Folder: Book Reviews.]. Owens was a national hero after the 1936 Olympics, but the climate of race relations in the United States made it difficult for him to profit on his accomplishment. He believed that the Black Power radicals had benefited greatly from the civil rights movement of the 1950s and 1960s and that their ongoing agitation was unfounded. (Thompson collection)

3. Record, Wilson. *The Negro and the Communist Party.* Chapel Hill: University of North Carolina, 1951. 340p. Review copy from publisher. Story of the 30 year effort of the Communist Party to channel African American protest in terms of Kremlin edicts rather than the Bill of Rights. After World War I, the Party chose blacks as a major target in its recruiting campaign. (Burns collection)

The Reconstruction Era (1863-1877)

1. Bennett, Lerone, Jr. *Black Power U.S.A.: The Human Side of Reconstruction, 1867-1877.* Chicago: Johnson Pub. Co., 1967. 401p. Announced in "Ebony Book Shelf," *Ebony*, January 1968, p. 20. Inscribed by the author to Thompson. For a brief period after the

Civil War, the first years of Emancipation, there was an upsurge of hope and achievement. "An understanding of this first Reconstruction is indispensable to an understanding of the second Reconstruction of the 1960s." (Thompson collection)

2. Du Bois, W. E. B. *Black Reconstruction in America*. New York: Atheneum, 1992. 746 p. Originally published as *Black Reconstruction* in 1935 by Harcourt, Brace. Annotated. Content: The black worker; The white worker; The planter; The general strike; The coming of the Lord; Looking backward; Looking forward; The transubstantiation of a poor white; The price of disaster; The black proletariat in South Carolina; The black proletariat in Mississippi and Louisiana; The white proletariat in Alabama, Georgia, and Florida; The duel for labor control on border and frontier; Counter-revolution of property; Founding the public school; Back toward slavery; The propaganda of history. (Dent collection)

3. Franklin, John Hope. *Reconstruction: After the Civil War*. Chicago: University of Chicago Press, 1962. 258p. Content: The aftermath of war; Presidential peacemaking; Reconstruction: confederate style; Confederate reconstruction under fire; Challenge by Congress; The South's new leaders; Constitution-making in the radical South; Reconstruction: black and white; Economic and social reconstruction; The era begins to end; The aftermath of redemption. (Burns collection)

Riots (urban)

1. Powell, A. Clayton, Sr. *Riots and Ruins*. New York: R.R. Smith, 1945. 171p. Annotations in the form of vertical line markings in margins. Content: Riot atmosphere; Touching off riots; Hoodlum's holiday; Responsibility; Clearing the ground for action; Three Vs; The right direction; Abolish discrimination; Democracy in action; A challenge and a compromise. (Burns collection)

2. Randall, Dudley. *Cities Burning*. Detroit: Broadside Press, 1968. 16p. A group of thirteen poems about the Detroit riots of 1967. (Dent collection)

3. United States. National Advisory Commission on Civil Disorders. *Report of the National Advisory Commission on Civil Disorders.* New York: Bantam Books, 1968. 654p. Announced in "Civil Disorders Report Flays," Jet, March 14, 1968, p. 8-9. Content: Profiles of disorder; Patterns of disorders; Organized activity; The basic causes; Rejection and protest: an historical sketch; The formation of the racial ghettos; Unemployment, family structure, and social disorganization; Conditions of life in the racial ghetto; Comparing the immigrant and Negro experience; The community response; The police and the community; Control of disorder; The administration of justice under emergency conditions; Damages: repair and compensation; The news media and the disorders; The future of the cities; Recommendations for national action; Supplement on control of disorder. (Thompson collection)

Notes

1. Gephi 0.8.2beta (Jan 03 2013). https://gephi.org/. [Last date accessed: 1/11/2014].

2. Hanneman, Robert E. *Introduction to Social Network Method*, Chapter 10: Centrality and Power. http://faculty.ucr.edu/~hanneman/nettext/ C10_Centrality.html [Last date accessed: 10/25/2013].

3. "Former Defender Editor, Ben Burns, dies at 86." *Chicago Defender*, February 3, 2000, p. 5.

4. Burns, Ben, *Nitty Gritty*, p. 184.

Index

American Daughter (Thompson), 19, 25n, 32-33, 39-40, 82-83
Artist and Influence, 8
Atlanta University Center, 1, 8

Baraka, Imamu Amiri, 24, 49, 78-79
Billops, Camille, 8
black bibliophiles,
 history of, 5-6
 types of, 6-9
Black Boy (Wright), 19, 30, 40
black collections in U.S. libraries, 1-3
Black World, see Negro Digest
BlackArtsSouth, 22, 24, 44, 46, 49, 52
Blockson, Charles, 2, 6-7
book collecting, 27-49
book reviewing, 29, 34-35, 46
Brathwaite, Edward Kamau, 46-48
Brooks, Gwendolyn, 39-41, 48-49, 71-72, 78
Bruce, John Edward, 7
Burkett, Randall K., 2
Burns, Ben, 2, 15-19, 27, 55-61, 64, 67-85, 87-88, 90-111, 112n

Callalo, 22, 45
Carnegie Foundation, 7
Chicago Daily Defender, 16, 19
Chicago Defender, 15-17, 19, 27-30, 32, 87, 100
civil rights, 15, 17, 22, 24, 30-31, 34-35, 40, 57-60, 62, 64-65, 69-71, 73, 77, 91, 93, 109
Clarke, John Henrik, 7, 11
Communist newspapers, 15, 29
Communist Party, 15, 18-19
Confessions of Nat Turner, The, (Styron), 23
Congo Square Writers' Union, 22, 24, 43-46, 49, 52

Dent, Tom, 2, 4n, 15, 21-25, 42-49, 55-64, 66, 68-103, 105-111
descriptors, most common, 56-57
Dick, Dakato, *see* Thompson, Era Bell
digital collections, 9-11
Du Bois, W. E. B., 1, 6-7, 11, 17, 21, 29, 76, 94, 110

Ebony, 2-3, 16-19, 21, 28, 30, 33, 37-38, 71, 72, 74-77, 79, 82, 86, 88-91, 96, 98-99, 100, 104, 109-110
Emory University, 8

Fisk University, 1
Free Southern Theater, 22, 24-25, 44-45
Freedomways, 7, 46, 52n

INDEX

George K. Hall Library, *see* Hall Branch Library
Gephi, 56-58, 67, 112*n*
Google Books Project, 9-10
Greenberg, Jack, 22

Hall Branch Library, 39, 41
Harlem Renaissance, 8, 21, 41, 81
Hatch, James, 8
HathiTrust Digital Library, 10
Heartman, Charles F., 1
Holte, Clarence, 1, 5-6
Houston Informer, 22
Howard University, 1
Hughes, Langston, 1, 8, 17, 21, 29-31, 35, 41, 43, 75, 77-79, 86, 107

integration, 15, 18, 20, 23-24, 96, 100-101

Jet, 2-3, 4*n*, 16-17, 34, 42, 72, 74-76, 80, 82, 86-87, 89-90, 94, 101, 103, 109, 111
Johnson Publishing Company, 3, 16-17, 19, 31, 33-35

Kgositsile, Keorapetse, 48

Library of Congress, 1
   Subject Headings, 55-57, 69

Marshall, Thurgood, 22
Motley, Constance Baker, 22
multiculturalism, 15, 20-21

National Association for the Advancement of Colored People, 17, 22, 86
Negro Digest, 2-3, 4*n*, 16, 19, 28, 30, 33-34, 73, 83, 98

Negro Society for Historical Research, 7
New York Age, 22
Negro Book Society, 35
Nkombo, 2-3, 22, 44, 48
New York Public Library, 1, 7

Penn State Library, 7
personal libraries,
   aesthetics of, 6
faculty research and, 6
Presence Africaine, 8

race mixture, 15, 17-18, 56
racial equality, 15, 17, 20, 22-23, 30, 72, 88, 108
racial identity, 15, 17, 20, 22, 23, 35, 44, 70, 96, 97
racist books, 2, 9-11
Randolph, A. Philip, 17
rare books, 1-2, 6-9
Reed, Ishmael, 24, 49, 53*n*, 78-79

Schomburg, Arthur A., 1, 5-7, 11, 12*n*
Schomburg Center, 9, 86
Sepia, 16, 30
Smith, Jesse Carney, 1, 4*n*
Southern Black Cultural Alliance, 22
Spingarn, Arthur, 1

Tan Confessions, 16
Temple University, 7
text network analysis, 55-111
   betweenness centrality, 64-65
   closeness centrality, 61-63, 69
   degree centrality, 59-61
Thompson, Era Bell, 2, 15, 18-21, 32-42, 55, 58-61, 64, 68-72, 74-111
Thompson, Portia, 8-9, 11

Umbra, 2-3, 24
Umbra writers workshop, 22, 24-25, 44, 49

Van Vechten, Carl, 1

White, Michael, 9, 11
White, Walter, 17
Woodson, Carter Godwin, 2, 4*n*, 6, 11, 17, 32
Work, Monroe, 11
Wright, Richard, 17, 19, 30, 38-41, 44, 84, 93

www.ingramcontent.com/pod-product-compliance
Lightning Source LLC
Chambersburg PA
CBHW022144160426
43197CB00009B/1426